FROM

Cocktail

TO

Chemo

MARY STOLFA

Acknowledgements

*First and foremost, I would like to thank God.
Without Him, I would not be here.*

*This book is dedicated to my Mom and Dad whom
I love very much. They are my heroes.*

*I would like to thank my wonderful parents and family for the
tremendous amount of love, support, and encouragement I
received—not only when I was sick, but each and every day:*

*Mom and Dad
Bernadette
Theresa, Mike, Michael, Daniel, Joseph, Julianna
Margaret, Stephen, Stevie, Gianni, Nicolette
Nicholas, Carol, John, Matthew, Grace
Ann Marie, Frank, Olivia, Diana*

*Since I was diagnosed back in 2001, the family has grown and I
am so very thankful to have every one of them in my life.*

*Thank you to every one of my special friends. I am truly
blessed to share my life with you. A very special thank you to
my dear friends Pam Wehrheim and Janine Ingardia.*

*Thank you to all of the great surgeons, doctors,
nurses, and technicians who saved my life.*

*Thank you to my fabulous editor, Joanne Shwed, for
her expertise and in bringing my book to life.*

*A special thank you to Elyse Trevers and Suzanne
Francis for their time in polishing my book.*

*Thank you to everyone who has touched my life and made me who I am today.
To all of the men and woman who have also fought the good fight and lost. To
those who won. To those who are still fighting. You are all my inspiration.*

—

Contents

CHAPTER 1

Too Young

I stood there, feeling paralyzed, as my father clutched me and squeezed tighter and tighter. My hands dangled at my sides; my shoulders were numb and limp. My head was buried in his chest, and I could feel his hands grabbing at my back as if he weren't able to hold me tightly enough.

"All I want you to do is live! Just live!" my father Ben cried out. I didn't utter a word as he shouted over and over, "You have to let it out and cry! *It's okay to cry!*"

I couldn't cry. I felt defeated.

Mary Ann, my mom, rushed in and pulled us apart. She tried to calm my father down, but he ran out the door. I turned around and walked over to my bed, lay down, and curled into a ball.

My body started shaking uncontrollably. I think I was going into shock. My mom lay down next to me, put a blanket over me, and then wrapped both of her arms tightly around me. Her body was nestled around mine. I could feel her trying to get closer to me, as if she couldn't get close enough. The more my body trembled, the tighter she'd squeeze.

I had breast cancer.

CHAPTER 2

Cancer Research

I was 11 years old. It was April Fools' Day 1984, and I was at my friend Suzanne's house around the corner. We dressed up in silly outfits and giggled as we made our way out the door. We headed up the block towards my house, discussing the "action plan" for the great joke we were about to play on my family.

We continued chuckling as we walked towards the front steps. I reached up and rang the bell. The door slowly opened and my sister stared back at us, but she wasn't laughing. She seemed very sad.

Looking down at me, she quietly said, "Mary, Grammy died. You'd better come in."

Suzanne and I looked at one another as my sister backed away and walked inside. Was that *her* April Fools' Day joke? We were young and naïve and didn't know any better. It sounds crazy but, at the time, I really thought that she might be lying.

Well, we weren't about to let her pull one over on us! We quickly agreed that Suzanne would wait for me at the corner down the block. If this were, in fact, some kind of joke, I'd meet her there in five minutes.

Was it that I didn't know any better, or was it that I didn't *want* to know any better? Looking back, I don't think I wanted to accept the fact that my grandmother was gone.

I slowly walked inside and closed the door.

The house was very still and quiet as I walked up the stairs and headed towards my mom's bedroom, where I found her crying. This was my mother's mother. My eyes were glued to the floor as I slowly walked into the room.

"I'm sorry about Grammy," I said ever so softly. I walked over to the bed and lay down next to her. Not many words were exchanged between the two of us; they didn't need to be.

After a while, I stood up and gazed out the window. I looked past the windowsill and stared at the trees in the backyard for what seemed like hours … thinking about the last time I saw Grammy Rizzuto.

Months before, my father stayed home with my sisters and brother, and my mom and I flew down to see Grammy in Florida where she lived with my aunt and uncle. She was very sick in the hospital.

The plane landed late that night, so we went to see her early the next morning. I waited outside of the room with my aunt as my mom went in with my uncle to see Grammy for the first time. After a while, they came out to get us.

My mom's eyes were watery and red as she wiped her nose with a tissue. My uncle took my hand, and the four of us walked into the room.

I couldn't quite reach her cheek to give her a kiss, so my uncle grabbed my waist and lifted me up. I reached over and gave her a gentle kiss on the forehead.

After he lowered me back down, I quickly pulled out a present for her that I was holding: a ceramic Cabbage Patch doll that I had painted from ceramic class especially for her. I raised it over the bed and held it high, waiting for her to take it.

She looked over at me from the corner of her eyes, too sick even to turn her head. There was a tube wrapped around her nose and ears. She had wires running out from under the covers to machines surrounding her bed. As her eyes met mine, she slowly lifted up one of her arms to reach for the doll.

Her hand was covered with bruises, and it had another one of those tubes attached to it, like the one around her face. As she reached for my present, she smiled at me. Her lips were caved in since she wasn't wearing her dentures. Under her breath, I heard her softly say how beautiful it was and how she loved it. My mom and uncle simultaneously lunged for the doll as it began to slip from her hand.

My Grammy was very special to me and I loved her very much. The two of us had a unique kind of bond, different from the rest of the grandchildren. I was a little fresh and maybe a tad bit more defiant than the others. She and I were both very stubborn where the other one was concerned, and we used to tease each other. She was relentless, and my uncompromising attitude always got us into trouble with each other.

She was often getting after me for something and, even as a child, I found myself getting after *her* for something as well. We'd never admit it, but we both enjoyed the special relationship we had.

Thinking back to the day of my communion at eight years old, I recalled one day when Grammy was in the bathroom with me and stood at the sink, rinsing out my new socks. I was playing outside with my friends earlier that day and company was coming soon. She wanted to freshen up the socks before everyone came over.

As I sat on the toilet seat beside her, I watched as she scrubbed and scrubbed my thin, silky, extra-long, dressy white communion socks. The moment the water, soap, and socks came together in her hands, they quickly turned slippery.

All of a sudden, I watched one of my beautiful new socks slide right out of her hands and straight down the drain! One minute you saw it; the next minute it was gone. Silence quickly filled the room, except for the running water.

Grammy stood there motionless, looking down at the sink, and her eyes began to glaze over. Maybe she was trying to figure out how it happened. Maybe she was thinking that it might come back up. Maybe—just maybe—she was praying that, in fact, it *would* come back up.

The little communion girl, who was sitting beside her, had just witnessed it all. I had seen everything from start to finish. She murdered my brand new sock with her own two hands, and she knew I'd point her out as the guilty party within seconds.

This wasn't just any old granddaughter. This granddaughter would take what Grammy had done wrong and run with it … *literally*.

With the other sock still dangling from the tips of her fingers, Grammy slowly shut off the water. She continued to stare at the empty drain but didn't risk the chance of looking over at me.

My jaw hung in astonishment. I slowly inhaled, filling my lungs with air, and my eyes opened, big and round and enormously wide.

At that very moment, I gasped in horror from what I had seen. From the look on my face, one would have thought that my *grandmother* had fallen into the sink and down the drain!

"Boy-o-*boy*, are you in trouble, Grammy ... *big* trouble!" I said, as I jumped up from the toilet seat and out the bathroom door. My pants were still down and sagging around my ankles. I tripped and stumbled as I ran through the house, shouting out for my mother. The words wouldn't come out of my mouth quickly enough.

"Mom! *Mommy!*"

After running around the house aimlessly, sliding into walls, tumbling, and picking myself up off the floor time after time, I finally found myself at the bottom of the stairs. My pants were still down and, by now, twisted tightly around my two ankles. I shouted up to my mother how Grammy had just washed one of my brand new communion socks down the drain!

You could see fear in my mother's eyes as she flew down the stairs towards all of the commotion, almost certain that something terrible had just happened.

"Can you *believe* what she did?" I continued to cry out.

Instantly, the house became very still and quiet, and a faint echo of laughter came from the bathroom ... it was my grandma.

I never met Suzanne back at that corner. My grandmother was 70 years old and died from ovarian cancer. The doctors said that she would have lived if she had been able to tolerate chemotherapy.

Grammy always said, "When it's your time to go, God will come and find you, no matter where you are or what you are doing." I guess April 1, 1984, was her time to go because God came and found her.

When she passed away, I wanted a little keepsake to remember her. My uncle sent some of her belongings to us in New York.

My mom handed me a crumbled brown paper bag and I went up to my bedroom to open it. I began to sob as I unfolded the top and looked inside. I put my hand deep down into the bag and slowly pulled out the ceramic Cabbage Patch doll I had given to her. She never had the chance to take it home from the hospital.

At that time, as an 11-year-old, in between *Woody Woodpecker* and *The Smurfs* on TV, I would hear public service announcements about "research" for a cure for this very bad sickness called "cancer." The only research I had ever encountered was when I went to the library to look up information in books or encyclopedias for an assignment my teacher gave me. If I needed answers, I would simply turn to the page that gave them to me.

Naturally, when I researched "cancer," I turned to section "C" in the encyclopedia. That was simple enough. At the time, I didn't think this "research" thing was as tough as everyone made it out to be.

The other kind of research I knew was about a scientist in a white lab coat, mixing boiling liquids from one glass tube to another. I even had a chemistry set, which I played with from time to time and took seriously. It wasn't always *play* for me.

After my grandmother's death, I thought that my experiments and concoctions might lead to big things. Hey, you never know, right? My mixture of salt, pepper, baking soda, and water might even turn into a medicine for that cancer.

After losing my grandma, I learned about this very bad sickness, which could take people whom I loved away from me. It wasn't like the sore throats or fevers I would get. It was the scariest sickness of all. I also knew that some bad-tasting pink medicine, like the kind I'd have to take from time to time, wouldn't make cancer better because, if it did, no matter how bad the taste, Grammy would have swallowed it to make her cancer go away.

During the following year after she passed away, I would often hear how money was needed to research a cure for cancer. I was certain that we needed to pay these "scientists" to go to the library or laboratory, or wherever they needed to go, to make a medicine so everyone with cancer could get better. It was too late for my Grammy now, but I didn't want anyone else whom I loved to go away.

I also knew that I had to tell as many people as possible. The more people who knew, the more money we could get; with more money, more scientists could do research. This would mean more of a chance to find a way to make everyone better who was sick.

As months passed, I thought about how I could get this money. At 11 years old, I considered opening up the Donald Duck bank on my dresser, but I didn't think that what it held—an old $2 bill, spare change, and useless coins I had collected over the years from our family trips—would make much of a difference.

I had to figure out another way. I knew that I didn't have enough on my own. Something else needed to be done ... something *big*. I was realizing that this "cancer" thing was bigger than everyone in my house. I set out on a mission although, at the time, I had no idea what I was about to do.

I decided to go to Mrs. Sheery, my principal's secretary. I requested a meeting with Mr. Hildebrandt, my principal, and asked if I could have an appointment as soon as possible.

"Mrs. Sheery, I need to discuss an important matter with him."

She smiled and penciled me in for the next day.

The following afternoon, I walked up to Mrs. Sheery with one of my friends. I held my clammy hands tightly together and asked her to let Mr. Hildebrandt know that I was there. A few minutes later, he came out and walked us back to his office.

I looked in awe across the tremendous wooden desk. He must have been at least 50 feet tall! Well, maybe not, but he sure looked that way after I sank down in my chair. It was as if we were in the White House and the President of the United States was sitting before us. It was extraordinary! I had never been in his office or even that close to him.

Mr. Hildebrandt's pipe holder was positioned on the side of the desk and, from the corner of my eye, I could see a fireplace off to the side. He sat in this beautiful leather seat behind his shiny wooden desk, with gold and expensive-looking trinkets perfectly positioned on it.

I was scared and intimidated but tried to remain focused. It wasn't about my wobbly knees and quivering voice. It was about finding a medicine—a cure—and getting the money to make that happen.

I was a determined sixth grader. A little shaky and a little shy, I sat down with my chin held high. Somehow, with great poise and confidence, I found the strength to present my request.

Mr. Hildebrandt sat quietly in his chair. His hands were placed in front of his chin and his elbows were leaning on both arm rests. He seemed casual, as if he were waiting for a request to install a snack machine in our lunchroom.

I cleared my throat, and my voice cracked as I apprehensively asked, "Um … Mr. Hildebrandt?"

I quickly looked over at my friend for reassurance and then down at the floor. At least 30 seconds passed and I repeated myself a little louder and more sternly than before. I looked directly into his eyes as I spoke.

"Mr. Hildebrandt? We need to cure cancer."

"I see."

He leaned forward, clearly taken aback, but maintained his composure. I continued.

"My grandma died from cancer last year. I wanted to help find a cure."

I could see a small smile through his fingers.

"So, how were you proposing to do this?" he asked.

I took a long breath and said, "I was thinking about putting on a show with the sixth graders. We could also sell greeting cards afterwards. The money we make could go to cancer research, so the same thing that happened to my grandma doesn't happen to anyone else."

I had somehow gained a little confidence, and continued.

"I was thinking that we could perform it on the stage in the gym ... that is, of course, if it would be okay with you? I promise that it won't interfere with anything. We can practice in the morning and afternoon, after school."

Without hesitation, Mr. Hildebrandt sat up in his chair and proudly said, "I think that is an absolutely *wonderful* idea, Mary!"

He stood up and shook my hand, and the deal was made.

Weeks later, after several practices and rehearsals, my friends and I gathered for a great performance. I pulled together most of the three sixth-grade classes in my school for an event to raise money for an extremely worthy cause—a cause, as I had explained to my principal weeks before, that was exceptionally important to me. The theme was "We Are the World."

We laughed, stumbled, and tripped all over the stage in front of an auditorium filled with teachers and classmates. It was a complete disaster, but it seemed to amuse my loyal and faithful elementary school. In fact, we videotaped the program and buried it in the school's "Time Capsule" for people to see many years later. Outside of the gym in the hallway, we also sold greeting cards.

At 11 years old, having just lost my grandma to cancer, I planned that show for a very special reason: We should use the money for one thing and one thing only ... *cancer research.*

That same year, my teacher instructed each member of our class to write a report on any subject. What did I choose? I cut letters out of white construction paper and glued C-A-N-C-E-R across the front of the folder. When you opened it, the index was scribbled with a marker on the first page: "Cancers from A to Z."

My book looked like an antiquated website, filled with information, charts, and educational statistics regarding all types of cancer. Page after page, cancer after cancer, it briefly described each one: bladder cancer ... brain cancer ... breast cancer. The last words I wrote on the breast cancer page (with many exclamation points) were, "And if you find a lump, do not wait! Make sure you get it checked out right away!"

I had the fundraiser, raised awareness, raised money, and gathered information regarding the disease so people could read and learn from it.

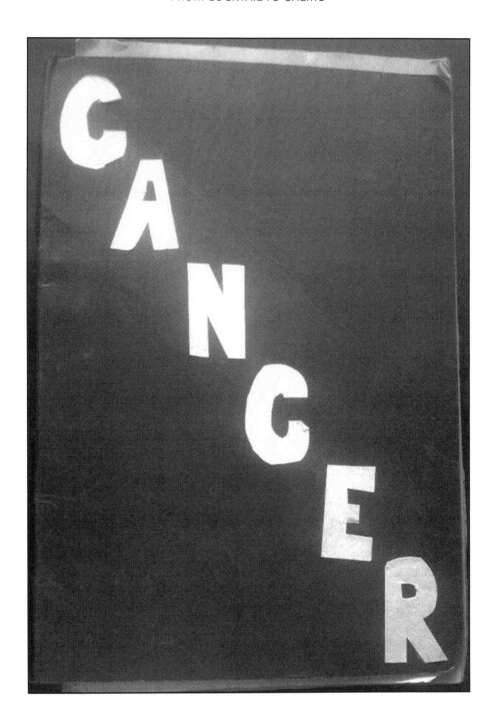

Even though I didn't raise millions of dollars, and my little report folder didn't reach thousands of people to educate them on cancer, it was the beginning of something ... but what?

"Why do boring research anyway?" my friends and I asked. "It's not like we're ever going to need them when we get older, right?"

The following year, when I was 12 years old, another tragedy struck my family. My other grandmother, Gram Stolfa, had gone for several tests, and we were waiting to hear from the doctors, who thought it was either colon cancer or pancreatic cancer. They told us that she might have a chance if it were colon cancer but, if it was in her pancreas, there wasn't much they could do.

Everyone was on edge for a week as we waited for the results, and it was devastating when we got the news. (I hadn't raised enough money to save my other grandma from cancer either.)

Gram lived with us in an apartment that my father built for her. I remember spending hours together while sewing, talking about her "era" and my "era," eating, cooking, and taking naps.

She'd tell me about her time growing up, and I would talk about how things were for me then. She'd show me how to sew on her sewing machine, and I'd show her the simple "hook and latch" sewing kit I got from the toy store.

Gram was always baking and cooking. I would sit at the kitchen table and watch as she'd repeatedly duck her head into the oven. She did it so often that her eyeglasses actually began to melt on one side and slowly became crooked! There were always some morsels of cookie dough or baking ingredients stuck on them. I loved to tease her about her "crooked cookie glasses."

After Gram's diagnosis, she became very sick, very fast. She knew that she didn't have much time left, so she decided to stay with my Aunt Nikki in Florida.

I stayed in Gram's apartment for the entire day before she left and even slept over that night. It was a very quiet, somber day and we did the same things we always did. We talked, laughed, napped, and ate every meal together. Neither of us said it, but we both knew it would be the last day we would ever spend together like that. The day went by ever so slowly, and we went to sleep early that night.

I clearly remember the morning she left for the airport. I was lying in bed very still, listening to her getting dressed and ready to leave. I kept my eyes tightly closed as I heard her zipper close her coat.

The floor beneath the rug creaked as she walked over to the bed where I was lying motionless. I felt her move the blanket away from my face as she kissed me several times on my cheek. I couldn't bring myself to open my eyes and look at her.

She tucked the blanket under my chin. I felt her hand stroke my hair several times and then slowly brush across my arm. I rolled my head to the side and buried my face in the pillow as she walked away. After she and my mom closed the door to the apartment behind them, I gradually lifted up my head. I listened to her and my parents talking as the front door slammed shut.

My grandma was gone. I dropped my head back down and sobbed.

Not long after that, my dad and some other family members flew down to Florida, one by one, to see her; they couldn't go at the same time. My mom's flight was scheduled after my dad came back. The night before she was going to leave, I begged my parents to let me go with her. I would do anything to see my grandma one last time.

We left together the next day and arrived at my aunt's house very late that night. We put our suitcases down and walked into the den, which had been set up like a hospital room.

After my mom kissed Gram, she brought me over to see her. A few seconds passed before I was able to lift up my head and look directly at my grandmother. The very first thing I noticed was that she didn't need those "crooked cookie glasses" anymore. Her eyes were gazing past me, staring directly towards the ceiling. I reached over and gave her a kiss.

I whispered, "Hi, Gram."

She couldn't say anything back, but I knew that she knew I was there.

For the week my mother and I stayed, I would sometimes help feed Gram. I remained fairly quiet as I spooned the food into her mouth. It was nothing like the times when we ate together back in her apartment.

Other family members were there visiting as well. The days passed by quickly, and it was finally time to go home. On the day we were leaving, when no one was looking, I walked over to Gram's bed. She was positioned on her side, facing everyone in the dining room. I took her arm and bent down to give her a kiss.

I whispered into her ear, "I love you, Gram."

We finished packing and left later that afternoon.

Not long after we were home, the phone rang in the middle of the night. A friend of mine was sleeping over and we were making our way down the stairs. My arms were full of pillows and blankets.

As the ring echoed through the house, I dropped everything and watched the linen tumble down the stairs. My head turned towards Gram's apartment and, at that very moment, I knew she was gone.

Eventually, her belongings were distributed amongst the family but, before anyone had a chance, I searched for the most important thing to me. I didn't want money, jewels, or any fancy belongings.

I looked through a couple of boxes and closets, and then made my way over to her dresser. I slowly opened the top drawer and found the only thing I needed, which was sitting on top of some clothing and handkerchiefs: her "crooked cookie glasses."

The following year, I went into eighth grade in junior high. A little older and a little more confident, I discussed my plans with Mr. Green, the vice principal. Once again, I gathered my friends to present a show. We performed two plays, which I had found in a children's book from the library.

We made the stage set out of cardboard and spray paint. We didn't have microphones and, in spite of many practices and rehearsals, had absolutely no direction and muddled our way through the entire show.

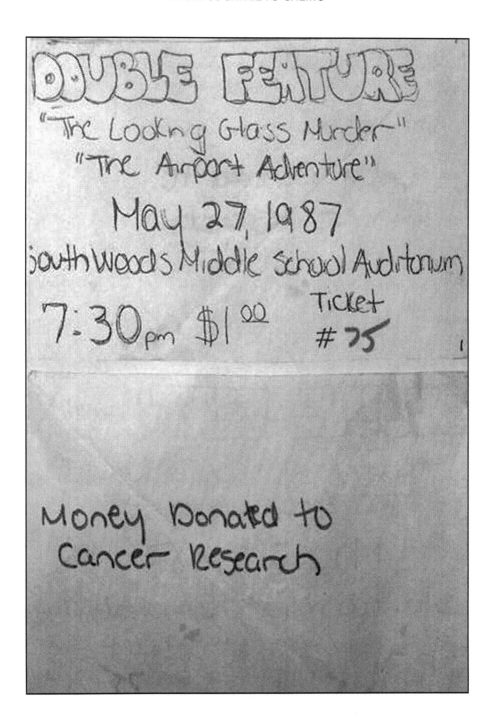

One particular act was supposed to take place at an airport. For that scene, I was the director as well as one of the performers. Before I stepped out in front of the audience, I cringed when I saw my friends prancing back and forth on stage. They were forgetting their lines and bursting out in laughter from the silliness of it all.

Then, it was my turn. I walked out and took center stage with a "show must go on" attitude. I was ready to pull it all together and save what was left of the show.

As I stood there, I was speechless. I watched in complete astonishment as my friends paraded across the stage, dressed in ridiculously crazy outfits. One after another, they would throw on hats, dresses, skirts, suits, and any other outrageous outfit they could find. Marching to and fro, they were cracking up with laughter as they walked past me.

While all of this was going on, suddenly and without warning, I saw the curtains begin to close … and open … and then close again. They swung back and forth in front of me and, at one point, even knocked me over! I looked out into the audience and saw everyone roaring with laughter. In spite of my embarrassment, the show was a tremendous success.

For weeks leading up to the performance, we had sold handwritten tickets to our families and to our friends at school during lunchtime. Each ticket stated that all proceeds would go towards … *cancer research.*

At the time, little did I know what would take place a decade and a half later. Sadly, that small amount of money that I raised for cancer research wasn't enough to help us find a cure because, at 27 years old, I was about to be diagnosed with breast cancer.

CHAPTER 3

Cheers!

G rowing up in an Italian household meant that, no matter how old I was, I always had a glass of table wine, Sambuca, or vermouth in front of me. Then, in my 20s, I discovered expensive wines and dirty martinis.

More than 10 years after the passing of my grandmothers, I was in my mid-20s and experiencing life to the fullest. I was still living at home, but I was respectful of my parents' rules. I would try to make as little noise as possible when coming home in the middle of the night; however, the sneaking didn't do much good most of the time. My dad would sometimes wait for me in the driveway with his robe, slippers, and a very unhappy face. My mom, on the other hand, would wait inside. I'd catch a glimpse of her feet, hanging off the side of the couch, just as my face popped through the front door.

At 24 years old, I knew exactly how to have fun and there were no holds barred. I frequented restaurants—upscale, downscale, five star, and dives with great food—throughout Long Island and Manhattan. I was wining and dining every other night, giving myself a day in between to recoup. At these dinners, I would often laugh so hard that, by the end of the night, it was difficult to hide the wine-induced purple teeth that resulted over the course of the evening.

However, purple teeth aren't as bad as a *blue tongue*.

One night, when a few of my friends and I were sitting in a Luxury Suite at an Islanders hockey game, I had somehow managed to finish off an entire bag of blue cotton candy. After going to the ladies room, I couldn't find my way back to our room, so I knocked on every door as I made my way down the hall. The courage one gains after a glass or two of wine is amazing.

Bang! BANG! *BANG!*

"Hello?" I said, as one of the doors opened.

The room was filled with men—all in black suits. They quickly invited me in, and I soon found myself sitting on one of their laps by the ledge, overlooking the stadium.

"Look! I ate a Smurf!" I said, as I shifted myself around and stuck out my blue tongue.

The nicely dressed man smiled and said, "Wow, you did!"

I looked over the edge of the partition at the players skating around on the ice, pointed downward, and smirked.

"I don't know very much about sports. Is the idea of this game for each team to score as many home runs as possible?"

The nicely dressed man started to laugh, just as I hopped up and off his lap.

"I'm Bobby," the man said, as he put his hand out to shake mine.

"Nice to meet you, Bobby!"

Just then, another man took my arm and escorted me over to the others. They were gathered around in a circle, just about to do a shot. We all took a glass off the tray, clinked them together, and then tossed the cocktail down our throats.

"I really do have friends, you know," I said to all of them as I swallowed. "They're over there." I pointed at a box on the other side of the stadium. "Hi guys!" I shouted, as I enthusiastically waved and tried to gain their attention. I could see my friends laughing, eating, drinking, talking, and looking everywhere except towards me. "My friends are right over there!" I repeated, as I waved and yelled across the arena.

"*Sure* you have friends," Bobby said.

After swinging both of my arms in the air, jumping up and down, and swaying back and forth, one of my friends finally noticed me. They began to grab at each other and point at me in disbelief. In sync and all at once, they *finally* waved back. I flew out the door and was somehow able to find the Luxury Suite fairly quickly.

When I walked back into our room, my friends said, "You were with Bobby Nystrom!"

I shrugged my shoulders and asked, "Who's Bobby Nystrom?"

At that time in my life, I didn't have a care in the world. I was flying to the Caribbean and cruising to the islands every chance I got. While in the Bahamas, I snuck away from friends who were sunbathing on the beach. The next thing I knew, I was strapped into a harness and parasailing over them, more than a thousand feet in the air. I waved and waved, but no one knew that the little colored dot so high in the sky was *me*.

Vacations usually consisted of relaxing in the sun, jet skiing, water skiing, horseback riding, shopping, and excursions; at night, we'd visit restaurants and clubs.

I never smoked cigarettes, but my friend Christine, who really didn't smoke either, tried to teach me one night when we came home from Senior Frogs, which was a local bar in Cancun. We hopped onto the bed and Christine lit a butt. She elegantly inhaled and exhaled.

Then, she handed me one of her Marlboro Lights and said, "Quickly inhale, like you're startled because *mommy's* coming."

I took the cigarette and did just that. After uncontrollably choking, I handed it back to her. We both chuckled as I continued to gag for the next few minutes.

"Let me try it again," I said.

I slid one of the cigarettes out of the cardboard box and put it in my mouth, acting like I was some sort of movie star. Then, I reached for the lighter. My thumb—with its long, fire-hazardous, freshly polished acrylic fingernail— slowly pressed down on the lighter switch. Just as the rigid wheel turned and the spark sprouted outward, my fingernail ignited. As I shook my hand, frantically trying to put out the flame, my pointer fingernail lit up.

After a few seconds, all five fingernails were in flames.

We both sat there and stared at the blaze, and then we giggled. No, we didn't call for help. We just sat there and uncontrollably laughed. We blew at it again and again but, the more we blew, the bigger the flame got. We finally managed to blow it out, and I was left unharmed. I decided then and there to leave my smoking days behind me!

When I wasn't setting my hand on fire, I was enjoying those vacations and sucking every bit of good out of life that I could get. I also went to concerts and shows in Manhattan as often as possible.

After going to a concert in New York City, my friends and I left the music hall, walked outside, and started to cross the street. I walked a few feet ahead as the others staggered behind me. Suddenly, I turned to the left and, out of nowhere, a taxicab came barrelling down the street. It came to a screeching halt and stopped directly in front of me. The cold steel pressed against my stomach, and both of my arms were draped across the hood of the car.

The cab driver screamed at me and waved his hands in the air from behind the dashboard. By now, my friends saw my body hugging the cab and rushed over. I peeled myself off of the car and the cab driver drove away. It was a miracle. My mom often told me that I kept my guardian angels on their toes, and she was right. After he left, I think that, if you listened closely enough, you probably could have heard a faint "phew!" in the distance.

At that time, I seemed to be jumping in front of taxis and ships. Towards the end of the night on a booze cruise, I hung over the front railing, arms stretched out to the sides, just like Leonardo DiCaprio and Kate Winslet in *Titanic*.

"I am the king of the world!" I shouted.

The captain announced over the loudspeaker that I needed to get down, but I still felt like I *was* on top of the world. There would be no stopping me now, I thought.

If I wasn't in front of a boat, I was seated in the back of a boat on my way to Fire Island to spend a few days at our summer rental house. A ferry would take us from Long Island to Fire Island on weekends. What a great summer that was! I was also much better on boats than on airplanes.

One time, my friends and I were leaving for a management seminar in Washington, D.C., and would soon be boarding the company jet. I bought a six-foot-tall bottle of wine that I thought would help ease our fear.

The plane was a six-seater.

19

After settling in from a rocky takeoff, I quickly dug out the cheap bottle of vino from behind the curtain at the back of the toy-sized airplane. I sat in my seat, buckled up, and placed the mammoth jug between my legs. Just as I began to twist the corkscrew, the pilot came over the loudspeaker.

"No alcoholic beverages are allowed on the company jet."

Surprised and disappointed, we all looked at one another as I pulled the bottle out from between my knees and forced it behind the curtain with the rest of the luggage.

When taking road trips with my friends, very little planning went into throwing bags of clothes and food into my car. We once drove down the eastern U.S. border, stopping at each state, and had one of the best times of our lives.

On another road trip with my friends Sue, Kate, and Kristina, we headed to Cape Cod. We arrived at Blueberry Manor, the bed and breakfast, fairly late that day. After Kate politely explained to the hosts that she didn't really like blueberries, we went to our rooms to unpack. We then changed our clothes and prepared for the evening.

Each night during our stay, we would go out for dinner and cocktails. Each morning, the hosts would start our breakfast by serving us fruit. By the third day, I was convinced that the fruit was making me sick to my stomach; of course, it wasn't the numerous dirty martinis I drank the night before!

One morning, the four of us walked down the stairs and sat around the breakfast table. The birds were chirping and the bright orange sun was coming through the many windows, shining directly onto the country wooden table. Warm muffins were placed on top of a plaid placemat.

Jan and Tom, our hosts, walked in from the kitchen with cheerful smiles.

"Good morning!" they both said.

As they made their way around the table, they placed a dish in front of each of us, which was filled with fresh fruit.

"Enjoy!" they said, as they walked back to the kitchen to prepare the rest of our breakfast.

I looked down at the plate, filled with bright melons, berries, and other succulent fruit. This morning would be different: I came prepared. I was not

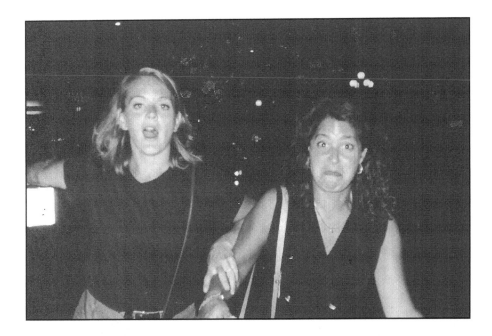

about to let the *fruit* make us sick again. I pulled out a plastic bag from my pocket and put my hands out towards my three friends in an effort to stop them from putting any of the fruit into their mouths.

"Wait!" I said. *"Don't eat the fruit!"*

I looked behind me. Jan and Tom were nowhere in sight, so I quickly poured my plate of fruit into the plastic bag and then turned to Kate.

"It's the fruit that's making us sick each morning. Give me your fruit!"

I made each of my friends pass me their fresh fruit, and I emptied their dishes into the plastic bag. I quickly handed back everyone's plate and tied up the bag. Just as Tom came walking in, I pulled my shirt over it and smiled.

"Wow! You girls must have loved the fruit! Would you like some more?"

By now, I was 26 years old and dating often. My friends were always setting me up with someone. I had a great outlook on life, and dating was just another one of my exciting adventures. I thought the worst that could happen is that I would make a friend, so I never passed up an opportunity to meet someone new. I felt that, when I least expected it and wasn't looking, I would meet my Prince Charming.

Sometimes, my friends would surprise me, and I would find myself out on an unplanned blind date. One Friday night, my friends Robin and Andy asked me to get together for drinks at the Garden City Hotel in Long Island. The three of us walked into the lobby. Andy and Robin spotted another girl and guy standing over to the side. They immediately smiled and we walked over to them.

"Mary, this is Peter. Peter, this is Mary."

I should have known—another setup! Peter—Andy's girlfriend's brother—was a New York City cop. They thought that we would be a perfect match. I put my hand out to Peter and he shook it.

"Nice to meet you, Mary," he politely said with a nervous smile.

Peter and I quickly hit it off. We began romancing, dating, and living life to the fullest: dinners, parties, stumbling into the house after a few cocktails, and falling into one another's arms. It took hours just to say good-bye at the end of the night. We kissed and hugged … and then hugged and kissed some more.

Life was great!

CHAPTER 4

A Moment in Time

It was Sunday night and I was lying in bed, chatting on the phone as I had done a hundred times before. It was late and the lights were off. The room was completely dark except for a glimpse of moonlight, which gleamed around the side of the window shade, and the bright digital numbers coming from the clock. Ann Marie, my friend since the third grade, and I were laughing and talking about the week we had.

"I know! Can you *believe* it?" I asked as we giggled like two teenagers.

I heard a knock on my door.

"Goodnight, Mary!" said my little sister Bernadette.

Bernie lives in a group home for mentally handicapped children during the week and comes home on the weekends. She is known as The Mayor at this school because of her popularity. No one can resist her overzealous and lovable personality. She wants a hug or kiss from everyone she meets, and that's exactly why everybody who meets her instantly falls in love.

My mom was in Bernie's bedroom across the hall, putting The Mayor to bed and getting teased by her. I continued to talk on the phone and go about my business, but I noticed a commotion outside my door. It was never an easy task putting Bernie to bed.

"Hold on for a sec," I said to Ann Marie. "Goodnight, Bernie. See you in the morning!" I shouted from my bed. "Listen to Mommy, or I'll have to come out there!"

"*Nooo*! I'll be good, Mary," the little liar promised.

Clearly in an effort to get on my good side, I heard a muffled "I love you, Mary" through the crack of my door. I presumed that she wanted to express her great love for me so I wouldn't be coming out of my room any time soon.

"I love you too, Bernie."

I continued to have a happy, lighthearted conversation with Ann Marie, just chatting for hours about nothing really important. During our conversation, I turned my head to the side and looked over at the clock. Inch by inch, I gradually raised my left hand to rub my left eye. As my arm came down, down, down, down, it *b-r-u-s-h-e-d a-c-r-o-s-s m-y c-h-e-s-t.*

It was as if the numbers on the clock came to a screeching halt, and time drew to a complete standstill. If it were a movie, it would be as if someone took the remote control, pointed it at me, and hit "slow motion." Our voices on the phone grew deeper and deeper as my arm began to descend one frame at a time.

At that split second, that instant, that precise frame, and *that very moment in time,* I felt a lump.

It felt like a small, hard pea. Being 27 years old, I never thought about doing self-breast exams; it never even crossed my mind. I didn't think it was necessary at my age.

My hand paused for a second, beginning to slightly tremble over the lump. As my body shuddered and I felt my muscles tightening up, I heard Ann Marie in the distance through the receiver.

"Mar? You still there? *Mary?*"

It sounded as if she were far away and speaking through a tunnel.

After a brief moment of silence, I quickly ended our conversation. I walked downstairs where I found my mother on the phone with my sister Theresa. Now, if anyone were going to panic, overreact, worry, and freak out about something (besides me, of course), it would be Theresa.

It probably wasn't in my best interest to turn on all of the living room lights and flash my breast at my mom while she was on the phone with Theresa, but I did. My mom jumped up from the couch and began doing a breast exam on me while holding the phone in between her shoulder and one ear.

Together, Theresa and my mom discussed my lump and had diagnosed me within minutes.

Theresa is like my worrisome second mother. Theresa and my brother-in-law Mike are like second parents. When I was little, I would always run to "Teesie" when I needed help. I may be a lot older now, but I still run to her when I'm in trouble.

While I was growing up, she was the first one I would go to for protection when everyone else in the house seemed to be chasing after me about something I did ... when she wasn't after me for something herself! That confidence and naughtiness may have gotten me into a lot of trouble when I was little, but that same defiance, stubbornness, and conviction would ultimately help me through what I was going to face in just five short months.

The next morning, Theresa was on the phone, making an appointment for me to see the doctor.

I thought I was in the prime of my life: partying, cocktailing, dating, vacationing, and dining.

I put it all on hold when one day I accidentally discovered a lump in my breast and went to check it out. My life wasn't going to change, and I was going through the motions like any other day.

It was a late September afternoon when I walked into Dr. Mazza's office, who was a gynecologist and a friend of the family. After a kiss hello and a few small pleasantries, the examination began.

The room was quiet. I could actually hear myself swallow.

Without hesitation, he quickly said, "It's nothing ... a harmless cyst," immediately dismissing it as if I had come to his office for a splinter.

My tense shoulders, constricted teeth, and clenched fists all relaxed as I let out a sigh of relief. The quiet examining room quickly filled up again with chitchat and laugher.

With a smile on my face, I walked out into the waiting room and told my mom the good news.

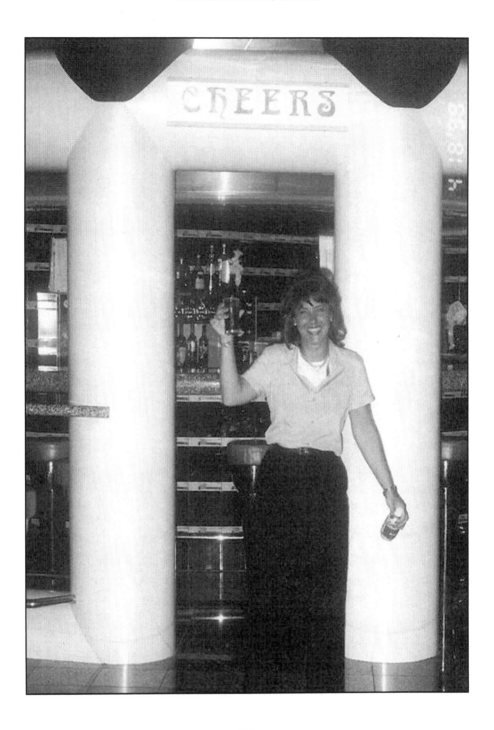

"He said it's nothing. See, Mom? I *told* you it wasn't anything to worry about," I continued to say as we got onto the elevator.

Twenty-seven-year-old women don't get breast cancer, right?

Gradually over the course of the next few months, the lump appeared to be growing. I actually felt it change from the feeling of a pea to a grape. My breast began turning colors—red and purple around the bottom—and even swelled a bit. Harmless cysts usually don't turn red and purple, do they? Then the pea, which turned into a grape, slowly began to feel like an orange.

Five months later, I found myself back at Dr. Mazza's office, explaining how the lump that was "nothing" seemed bigger. This time, I didn't take my mom along for the ride; instead, I insisted on going to the doctor all by my brave self. In a million years, I didn't think it would be something so bad. I decided to leave everyone at home so they wouldn't worry. I figured that the doctor would examine me and, once again, he would send me on my merry way.

I truly trusted Dr. Mazza because we had known him for years. Again, after a kiss hello and some small talk, he nonchalantly stretched his arms out and started whistling as the examination began.

The second he placed his hands on me, I knew that something was wrong. My friendly, laid-back doctor suddenly became very agitated and serious. His face turned pale. With a look of terror in his eyes, he gazed past my shoulder and stared at the jar of sterile gauze pads and tongue depressors. He immediately sent me to another office for a mammogram.

I was still thinking, "*Cyst*? It's definitely a cyst."

Cancer was the furthest thing from my mind and, surprisingly, I still wasn't very alarmed. In fact, I had plans for dinner later that evening, and my first thoughts were how this test was going to interfere with my social time.

I agreed to get the mammogram—not that it took much coaxing. This would be my first mammogram.

Once I got to the office, I put on a hospital gown and a very nice technician walked me down the hall and escorted me into another room, which was dimly lit with one fluorescent light. A tall machine stood in the right-hand corner of the room with an empty chair a few feet away.

I pulled my gown down on my left shoulder, stretched up onto my tippy toes, and lay my left breast on top of the plate. The technician walked over and moved my breast up, down, left, and right—and in directions that I didn't know were possible!

I caught a glimpse of her leg through the glass plate between my boob and her arm. It actually looked as if it were rising up into the air to gain momentum. After a brief pause, her foot crashed onto the gas pedal below and the other half of the plate came down. She pressed the pedal again and again, as if she were competing in a race-car competition. If I listened carefully enough, I bet I could have heard someone outside the room, firing a gun into the air and saying, "On your mark, get set, go!"

This nice technician, who suddenly turned masochistic, was definitely heading for the finish line.

"Are you okay?" she asked.

"Sure. I'm okay," I blurted out in agony.

The tech ran to the other side of the room, behind the glass window.

"Okay, honey. Hold your breath and try not to breathe. Okay, sweetie?"

As if pain weren't enough, she would do me in with oxygen deprivation.

"Make sure you hold your breath. Okay, darlin'? We wouldn't want to have to start all over again, love."

Now a threat? Pain and suffocation wasn't enough? We needed threats?

After finishing, she walked me back to the examining room and wished me luck with everything. She said that she was surprised to be giving someone my age a mammogram.

As she closed the door behind her, I settled into the chair and waited with bated breath, trying to listen to the doctors and technicians in the next room discuss my films. I bent forward with my ear as close to the door as possible. I was holding my gown closed as I tilted my chair towards the crack of the door.

It was an unsteady balance, leaning on only two of the four chair legs, but it gave me the advantage of getting closer to the door while still remaining seated in the off chance that someone unexpectedly walked in. In this way, I could easily tip back, keeping my innocence intact. I was up to no good, but no one would be the wiser. Sometimes, I'm just too damn clever for my own good.

I stopped chewing my gum during the brief moments they spoke, so I could better listen to what they were saying. I didn't seem to be getting very far in my efforts to hear through what appeared to be a steel, double-padded, triple-plated, airtight, soundproof, bulletproof, freaking eavesdropping-proof door.

Since it wasn't going very well for Angela Lansbury (me), I decided to lean forward just a *tiny bit more*. I suddenly heard voices getting closer. They must be walking towards me! I quickly tipped the chair back in place, utilizing my shrewd and ingenious plan, but, as I came down … *slam* … I landed on top of my foot.

"Ouch! *Dammit!*"

I quickly jumped up, causing my gown to fly wide open. Everything popped out as I nervously looked down. I could hear the doctors and technicians' voices getting louder and louder as they approached the door. With both hands, I grabbed the sides of my gown and quickly pulled it closed.

I imagined a voice through the intercom: "Beware: Mad Flasher in Exam Room 3." I shifted my chair back, wrapped my gown around the front, and settled down as two of the technicians walked in. Why couldn't they have spoken just a *little* louder? I would rather know what was going on before they told me. I never liked surprises.

They told me that the mammogram was inconclusive, and I would need to have a sonogram. They led me into another room and told me to lie down on the table.

Doctors and technicians walked in and out. One by one, they took hold of this long instrument with a sticky Vaseline-like substance dripping from the end, circled it around my breast, and gazed at the monitor propped beside me. Each person wore the same bewildered face when he or she looked at the screen.

Since the entire bottom of my breast was purple, one of them asked me if I had recently bruised myself.

"Nope," I answered, still not very alarmed.

"Can't they hurry this?" I thought. "I have to get home to shower before going out for dinner."

After the sonogram was finished, they told me to go back to Dr. Mazza's office. I drove back there and they immediately called me inside. He looked extremely worried and told me to have a seat.

"Do you think it's anything bad?" I asked.

Einstein was finally beginning to worry.

I'd always worry about things that never ended up happening. I'd torture myself over the stupidest things in life. Was I not nice enough to this person? Is that person mad at me because she didn't smile?

How many times had I gone to the doctor in the past for a sore throat or cold, and convinced myself that I had pneumonia or meningitis, or sprained my leg and immediately pulled out old crutches because I was certain it was broken? Give me a temperature of 101 and I'm suddenly dying of scarlet fever. Itchy, watery eyes? Must be some rare form of eyeball disease. For some reason, I always seemed to skate past the minor diagnoses like, um, *allergies*?

Okay, so I overreacted once or twice in my life but, for things that *did* happen, I never seemed to anticipate them. Heck, throw a lump in my breast and I agonize over dinner plans!

I didn't think about a small lump leading to such horrible possibilities. This was the first time *I didn't think the worst*, and it was the worst that was about to happen.

"Well, we just want to make sure." Dr. Mazza said, as he shuffled through his Rolodex.

"Make sure of what?"

As he began dialing the phone, he told me that he wanted me to see a surgeon right away. After calling a couple of them, he got me in to see Dr. Derini. (You will soon see why I call him "Dr. Angel.")

"I want you to see him tonight, okay?" Dr. Mazza said.

My mom and dad kept calling my cell phone to find out what was happening. Remember, I had banned everyone from coming with me that day. I insisted on going to the doctor all by my brave self. Well, my brave self decided that it was now time for Mommy and Daddy. They said they would meet me at the surgeon's office.

Who knows how long we sat in the waiting room, but it was late and dark outside. The jam-packed waiting room eventually cleared out and the last patient finally left; only my parents and I remained.

"Mary Stolfa?" the nurse called.

She introduced herself as Dawn, Dr. Derini's head nurse. She escorted the three of us into Dr. Derini's back office. As we walked in, I looked around the room in awe. I took a seat closest to the window, and my mom and dad sat next to me.

The entire room was filled with angels: angel figurines, angel plates, angel dolls, and angel pictures. It was incredible! Each piece tied into the next, almost united, giving the appearance of massive wings stretching from one wall to the other.

I looked around at the individual angelic faces, and it seemed as if they were looking back at me. Had God sent me His angels?

Dr. Derini was like an angel himself. If I didn't know better, he might have had wings tucked under that suit of his. He had a gentle, pleasant face and a kind, compassionate personality to match.

I remember sitting beside my parents. As nervous and frightened as I had finally become, I didn't want to let them see how I was feeling. If they didn't see me worried, maybe they wouldn't worry either. *Not a chance.* They looked as if they were being held at gunpoint.

Dr. Derini walked me over to the other side of the room by the wall with the x-ray screen. He flipped on the switch and put my x-rays up against it. I stared at the large, white mass on the picture of my breast.

He pointed at the x-ray and told me that, although he wasn't absolutely certain what it was, he *was* absolutely certain that he wanted it out. We scheduled a lumpectomy for the following Monday.

He wrapped his arm around me and told me that everything was going to be okay. I looked up at him, back towards the angels, over to my x-ray hanging on the wall, and then back down to the floor. We all walked out of the office together. As the three of us left his office, we did not utter a word.

It doesn't have to take a year to change a person's life. It doesn't have to take a week, a day, or even an hour.

All it takes is one simple moment.

CHAPTER 5

Draw

Months before I discovered the lump, I found myself tired constantly, needing to take naps before I went anywhere. I thought I was just a little run down.

"Maybe I'm going out too much and overdoing it," I thought. "Maybe that's why I'm so tired and not feeling very well."

I had made plans to go out with family and friends the Saturday night following my visit to Dr. Derini. It was two days before the lumpectomy and everyone wanted to take my mind off the upcoming surgery. I took a nap before getting dressed, as I had become accustomed to doing.

Peter came to pick me up on Saturday night and we went to the bowling alley to meet our friends. I bowl horribly, but it was fun swinging that huge bowling ball in between my legs with both hands to gain momentum, and then throwing it down the lane … in some cases, *two lanes*! Real competition never crossed our minds. It was just good, old-fashioned fun with family and friends.

I had an innocent kind of fun that night: enjoying the good things that life had to offer and realizing the simplicity of it all. I didn't think of what the future might hold. I never thought about being bald. I just tucked my long hair behind my ear when it fell in front of my face as I bent down. I also didn't think about being left with just one breast. Like any other girl, I picked up my bra strap when it fell off to the side of my shoulder.

I put a big, glowing smile on my face, which was a bright shade of purple from the wine, and enjoyed the night with everyone around me. Mastectomy, tests, tumor, chemo, cancer, and dying were thousands of miles away but, little did I know, they were all quickly approaching.

Here I was, though, tossing the bowling ball down the lane and thinking that we were all out to have a good time since I'd be laid up in bed for a few days. I was probably the only one that night who was thinking of my surgery as simple. I could see the look in their faces and actually feel the vibes.

I went on with the night and had a great time. I drank too much, bowled too much, laughed too much, and, when it came time to say goodnight to everyone, I didn't realize how much I loved life too much. Within days, I'd be fighting for this great life of mine.

The following Monday morning, I lay on the operating table, trying to control my teeth from chattering and my body from trembling, but I couldn't stop either. Technicians were hooking me up to all sorts of machines.

Dr. Derini walked in and smiled at me. My eyes welled up with tears as he clutched my left hand. My other arm was positioned straight out in the other direction. He squeezed tightly and asked how I was doing.

"I'm okay," I muttered while trying not to cry.

He continued to look down at me with a warm smile and firmly held my hand. From the corner of my eye, I could see the anesthesiologist inject something into my other arm. My eyes slowly began to close and I went to sleep.

I woke up groggy from the lumpectomy, and the nurse asked if I wanted her to get my mom and dad. I nodded "yes." Before long, they both came in to see me. After a short time in the recovery room, I was able to leave.

Peter and the rest of my family greeted me when I got home. The week went by slowly as I recuperated. It was quiet because I didn't tell most of my friends that I was having surgery so I wouldn't worry them; however, I spoke with the few I did tell. I still hadn't heard from Dr. Derini's office regarding the pathology report, but I wasn't very anxious about getting the results.

When my parents went out for even a short period, they'd call again and again, asking whether the doctor had called. I remember teasing them about making such a big deal. This was so unlike me, but I just wasn't thinking the worst.

I was relaxing at home, away from work, and enjoying a mini vacation that actually wasn't half bad! Hey, a little operation for a week off? I'll take it! Anesthesia or work? Work or anesthesia? It's a tough call. In fact, if it were summertime, I just might have slapped on some baby oil and soaked up a little sun.

Maybe I used up all my worry, or maybe I had worried so much and so often about things that never took place that I couldn't fathom the thought of something so bad *actually* happening.

To add insult to injury, I even joked about the entire situation with friends. I was talking on the phone with my friend Kate. We chuckled, giggled, and even snorted over a story another friend told us. To this day, I'm still not sure if the story is true, but we seemed to have a pretty good laugh over it.

It was about a woman who had a tumor removed. When she came out of surgery, the doctor told her that the benign tumor had hair growing out of the top and teeth coming out of the side!

Kate joked, "Can you imagine, Mary? Would you rather have a malignant tumor or a tumor with hair, teeth, eyeballs, and a nose?"

"Ha! I'll take the malignant tumor!" I cried out with laughter.

Well, I guess you had to be there because it was funny at the time. I rolled over in my bed and we continued laughing about the many types of funny tumors there could be.

I was recovering well. At the time, the chances of a cancerous tumor in a woman under age 30 were 1 in 20,000. I couldn't imagine that, out of a 20,000:1 chance, I would draw the cancer card.

The following Thursday, my friend Lisa asked me to go to dinner with her and her mom. It had been three days since the lumpectomy and I hadn't been out of the house. They picked me up and we went to a local Italian restaurant. It was great to be out, wining and dining again!

After eating, drinking, and having some great laughs, I came home and was getting ready to go to bed. I put my leftovers in the refrigerator and walked up the stairs to my bedroom. I carefully changed into my pajamas since I was still sore, and then played back the messages on my answering machine. I grabbed the remote and flipped on the TV.

As I began settling down, the telephone rang. I looked over at the clock: 8:22 p.m.

"Hello?"

It was cancer, calling to tell me that I drew the winning card.

My legs went numb. I grabbed onto my treadmill to keep myself from falling down.

"Oh, my God. I have *cancer*," I mumbled to myself.

I thought I heard wrong.

Dawn, from Dr. Derini's office, slowly repeated herself. The doctor was away, so she was calling for him with the results of the pathology report.

"What? Did she just say it *wasn't* cancerous?" I mumbled again.

"Mary, I am so sorry to have to tell this to someone so young. The biopsy results show that it *was* cancerous."

I was speechless.

"Are you okay, Mary? Dr. Derini wants you to come in Sunday to discuss everything in detail. Do you think you'll be able to come in?"

I still didn't answer.

"You know, we really don't know the extent of it. He may have even gotten most of it out already."

"Okay, okay. Thank you very much, Dawn," I blurted out.

My entire arm was shaking as I clenched the phone and pressed it firmly against my ear. I started trembling so violently that my hand actually began knocking the receiver repeatedly against my lip.

Dawn asked, "Do you have someone home with you?"

"Yes, yes, I do. My mom and dad. Thank you very much for calling, but I'd better go now."

I wanted to get off the phone. My body was shivering from head to toe. I don't remember the rest of the conversation, but I do know that it didn't last very long.

I dropped the phone out of my hands and stood motionless in the middle of my bedroom. I was still clinging to the treadmill bar as I looked down and saw my legs violently shaking through my pajama pants. There is no other way to describe the feeling I had other than pure terror.

"What do I do now?" I thought.

I looked over at the door and heard my mom across the hall in my sister's room, making her bed.

"How can I possibly tell my mother and father that I have cancer?"

It sounds unbelievable but, for a split second, I actually thought about lying to them. I thought about telling them that everything was okay. Thousands of thoughts ran through my mind within a matter of seconds. Cancer to me wasn't an illness; it was a death sentence.

I continued staring at the door for some time and listened to my mom making her way around my sister's bedroom. I heard her walk back and forth from the linen closet and then to her room. As I listened, my heart sank deeper into my chest.

I felt faint as I put one shaky leg in front of the other and gradually made my way to the door. With each unsteady step, my legs wobbled from side to side. I grabbed hold of the TV stand, dresser, and desk, and then lunged for the doorknob. I wrapped my hands around it and slowly turned the knob.

As the door opened, I lifted my head up and caught my mom's eyes. I was seconds away from breaking her heart, and I knew it. It killed me to have to do it.

She was holding a pile of blankets in both hands as the words just fell out of my mouth.

"Mom … it's cancer."

She stood there stunned, staring back at me in disbelief.

My head dropped down as I backed into my room. The pile of blankets she was holding fell to the floor as she ran to the top of the stairs, screaming for my father. I couldn't hear what my dad was saying, but my mom raced down the stairs.

I didn't know what to do with myself. All I knew was that my parents were incredibly devastated, and I was the one responsible for it.

I almost fell into a trance. I collapsed to the floor, reached for the phone, and called Lisa. She, too, was in shock.

"Let me come over right now," she said.

"No, no. It's okay. I'd better go. My parents are upset. Good-bye."

One of the hardest things I've ever had to do was to tell my parents that I have cancer; telling family and friends was the next worse thing. I felt as if it were somehow my fault. I was the one who went and got cancer. What happened? An hour ago, I was laughing my way through dinner. It is truly amazing how a person's life can be changed instantaneously.

I began making every plea to God and offering any deal with Him imaginable. Like many people faced with something over which they have no control, I began promising the sun, the moon, and the stars.

"Please, dear God, I beg You! I promise I won't complain about anything anymore. I won't … I swear, I won't. If I can just go back in time to be grateful for every good thing that ever touched my life, I will. If You'll just give me one more chance, I'll be thankful for all the blessings You've given to me. I promise. Please just make this all be one bad dream!"

I remember thinking how it might really be a dream, such as ones I've had in the past—dreams so real that you actually wake up laughing or crying. I thought that, at any minute, I might wake up. Even better, Dawn would call back to tell me that she was wrong.

As I sat on the floor in the middle of my bedroom, my phone rested quietly beside me. No one was calling to tell me that it was all a big mistake. I wasn't going to wake up any minute to find that it was all a bad dream. It was too late for promises.

I had cancer.

The news spread fast. Within the next hour, everyone seemed to find out and insisted on coming over. All I really wanted was to be by myself.

My friend Ann Marie started crying.

"Don't worry," I consoled her. "It's no big deal."

I called Lisa back, asking her to call my sister Margaret to try to make her feel better because there was dead silence on the other end of the phone when I spoke to her. I didn't want anyone getting upset on my account.

The house spun into a whirlwind, like a tornado grabbed hold of it and whisked it into the air. It was all spinning round and round—people, thoughts, fears, and my life—in an uncontrollable circle.

At about midnight, everything finally began to quiet down. My parents were in their room, and all of the lights in the house were off. I opened my bedroom door and quietly walked down to the kitchen. The nightlight my mom kept on above the counter was the only light in the room. I was barely able to make out the side of the kitchen table from the hallway.

I walked towards the kitchen table and continued around it without stopping. Alone in the dark, I paced around the table. I must have circled it at least 100 times that night, just imagining how my entire body was probably filled with cancer and that I might not make it through the night.

This was the hand I was now being dealt, but I couldn't remember asking to play. I didn't place a bet. My cards weren't an ace or a king or a queen or a jack.

I drew cancer.

CHAPTER 6

Chance

Pandemonium ensued at my house from the Thursday I got the news until I went to Dr. Derini's office the following Sunday. We met to discuss my results and what needed to be done. As my parents and I sat across the desk, Dr. Derini explained how cancer works. He slowly folded his hands together and reached towards us.

"Everyone falls into different sides of the spectrum."

He positioned his arms directly in front of us to signify the spectrum.

"Some people fall all the way to the left," he said, as he swayed his left hand to the side, "and some fall to the right." His right hand shifted in the other direction. "Some fall in the middle," and he nodded his head forward.

I'll never forget those words. It was his way of telling us how every individual can be different. Some survivors go into remission for a time; unfortunately, and for some inexplicable reason, some do not survive. I already knew that.

I could not believe that this man was actually sitting there and telling me that I could die. I can't die. He doesn't know what he's *talking* about! I believed that Dr. Derini was trying to be as gentle as possible. It was his job to explain this frightening and cruel disease, as difficult as it may have been for him.

He looked directly at me, straight into my eyes, made a tight fist, and swung it in the air.

"We only have one chance to *really* knock this thing out and get rid of it for good."

One chance? That's all? What if we miss it?

He recommended a mastectomy, and then most likely chemotherapy and radiation. He also wanted me to go for full body and bone scans to make sure the cancer hadn't spread.

Spread?

"Does he think it has already spread?" I thought. This can't be happening!

From the corner of my eye, I glanced at my parents to my left. They both looked as if someone had zapped them with a stun gun. They were just staring at him.

Then, I saw my dad looking around and becoming very anxious. He started rubbing his eyes and then his head. Over the years, a vein that ran across my father's temple to his forehead would protrude when he became upset. This same vein made a pulsing appearance now; I knew that look all too well.

I remember that look when I was six years old. That vein looked like it was ready to burst out of my father's head as he asked me who scratched the side of his brand new car—a rhetorical question, of course. He already knew that the handlebar on my bicycle swiped across it earlier that day. He was just asking so, after committing murder, he already had a confession.

As my dad began to get upset and squirm in his chair, I turned my head to the side, just enough to see my mom's hands beginning to turn white. Her pocketbook was sitting on her lap and she was squeezing the straps so tightly that she must have cut off the blood to her hands.

I couldn't believe that this was happening, and I couldn't believe that I was doing this to them. My mom and dad have done everything for my family, and now I was putting them through something so terrible. *They didn't deserve this.*

I could not have asked for more wonderful parents than my mother and father. They are the epitome of what every child looks for in a parent. My three sisters—Theresa, Margaret, and Bernadette—and my brother Nicholas have all learned from my parents' example how to be caring, loving, understanding, trusting, encouraging, courageous, and patient. If I can one day be even half the parent that my mom and dad are, I will be extremely blessed.

They taught us the difference between right and wrong, how to make the right decision with difficult choices, to try our best to succeed, and that, if failure ever crosses our path, how to accept it with dignity and learn from it. They've always said that it's okay to fall, just as long as we get back up and try to walk again.

Their lessons of judgment and wisdom would ultimately help decide my fate. I needed to be strong and make all the right decisions. I knew that there wasn't room for failure or error with this situation. Every choice I'd make from this point on would have to be the right one.

What was I going to do with all the information Dr. Derini was giving to me? This was completely out of my league.

"I'm just 27 years old!" I kept thinking.

Gently, he continued to explain everything to us while being detailed and kind at the same time.

Well, at least I *think* he was. I'm not quite certain because I stopped listening after the body scan part. At that point, none of us were saying very much. We were completely mesmerized. Then, Dr. Derini began discussing the results of the pathology report.

Okay, Dr. Derini … English translation, please! The only thing I really understood was the fact that I had cancer, people die from cancer, and now I was probably going to die from cancer. That's it.

Before we left his office, he handed me a pink folder containing a list of support groups and other information. He told me that a girl named Jesse, who was about my age and who had been sick as well, would call me.

With false assurance, I thanked Dr. Derini, told him that I was okay, and then led my parents out the door. I particularly remember leading because I wanted to show them how strong I was by keeping my head up and my shoulders back—like a soldier; however, there was an inexplicable tension in the air, as if the three of us would instantaneously collapse all at once if just one of us fell apart.

Without a word, we walked out of the building and into the car. I sat in the back seat, and my dad turned out of the parking lot and headed home. We rode in complete silence. I think the grief we all felt was almost unbearable. No words could have given it justice. Little by little, the fear I tried so hard to bury slowly began to surface.

When we finally arrived at home, I walked in the door and immediately headed upstairs to my bedroom. After I took off my coat and lay it on the chair, my father walked into the room.

He threw both of his arms around me and starting screaming. My mom rushed into the room and pulled us apart, and my dad ran off to his bedroom. I walked over to my bed to lie down, and my mom followed and wrapped herself around me. I was trembling uncontrollably.

A few minutes later, and not knowing any better, my sister Bernie walked in. My mom jumped up and, despite her attempt to take Bernie out of the room, she was able to make her way over to me. She bent down and gave me a kiss. I remained motionless as one tear after another dripped down the sides of my face. My pillow was becoming soaked as I stared ahead at the wall on the other side of the room.

Everything was a blur, but I remember barely making out my sister's innocent face as she stood over me and smiled. Although mentally handicapped, she still knew that something was wrong and needed to make it better. Bernie made every attempt to comfort me by smiling, kissing, and hugging. My mom was finally able to grab hold of her hand and lead her out of the room.

I heard a commotion downstairs. My brother Nicholas and sister-in-law Carol had come over. I could always go to my big brother Nicholas for help and advice, but there wasn't much help or advice he could give me now.

The bedroom door slowly opened, and I remember seeing my sister Margaret and brother-in-law Stephen walk into the room. I buried my face almost completely in the blankets as I continued to sob quietly. It wasn't a typical kind of crying. The muscles in my face and throat were numb because my face was frozen into a catatonic daze.

My eyes were filled with tears, so my vision was blurry and I wasn't able to see very clearly. Both Margaret and Stephen looked as if they were standing in front of one of those warped mirrors at a carnival. Their faces stretched down to the floor and their bodies distorted.

They each seemed to have the same look of terror on their faces as they reached over and kissed me. I didn't know what they were saying because everything sounded muffled. My mouth hung open like a scream, but no sound came out.

I knew I was in for the fight of my life. There would be no do-overs. I would have just *one chance.*

CHAPTER 7

No Rules in the Game of Cancer

By the next day, my father was making countless phone calls, including one to schedule the required scans. I was extremely anxious and wanted to get them done. Suddenly, every organ in my body was hurting.

"Must be the cancer," I thought.

I figured that the cancer had spread and it was already too late.

Dawn, from Dr. Derini's office, called to see how I was doing. She gave me her home phone number in case I needed her for anything. She was wonderful and said that everyone at the office was asking about me.

Later that morning, I knew it was time to tell Peter. He needed to know. I didn't have the heart to tell him in person, so I called him on the phone.

"Hi Peter," I quietly said. "How are you?"

"I'm fine."

After I made small talk and beat around the bush for a bit, he knew that something was up. It wasn't easy, but he was finally able to pry it out of me.

"The results came back from the biopsy," I said. "It's cancer."

"What else?" he blurted out. "*Tell* me!"

It was as if the next words out of my mouth were going to be "… and I only have one month to live …"

I caught him off guard and could hear him beginning to breathe more heavily. He stuttered nervously for a few words, unable to articulate a complete sentence.

"Let me … come … over!"

"I'll be fine," I said. "Don't worry."

Over the next 20 minutes, I was unsuccessful in reassuring him. He reluctantly hung up the phone after I insisted that everything was going to be okay.

Later that night, he came over. We drove to a small, private beach. It was a cold March night, and we bundled up and walked arm in arm towards the water.

In the past, I would go there to collect my thoughts. I led Peter towards several huge boulders. As a teenager, I would jump up onto these big rocks and talk to God. It was one of my special places.

The sky was clear as we both leaned back and looked up. The stars were shining brightly against the deep blue midnight sky. Peter wrapped his arms tightly around me and pulled me close.

"No matter what happens, Mary, we're going to go through this together, okay? It's not going to be easy, but I'm going to help you."

After that, we didn't say very much and just held onto one another tightly.

The next day, my mom, my dad, Peter, and I went for my magnetic resonance imaging body scan. For days, I had been waiting impatiently to go for several tests to make sure the cancer was contained to just my breast.

My eyes welled up with tears as I lay on the table. The MRI technician inserted an intravenous line into my arm to infuse dye, which would contrast any abnormalities, and immediately grabbed my hand and squeezed it firmly.

"Don't you worry," she said warmly. "I was diagnosed many years ago with cancer and I'm a survivor!"

The table began to roll slowly into a big, round, closed-in tube. My nose was so close to the top that it almost pressed against the machine. All through the test, I heard a lot of noise around me— bang, *bang*, BANG!—like someone striking a hammer against the side. If I heard a delay between any of the thumps, I got extremely nervous because I thought that they saw something and had stopped to look at it. Finally, it was over, and the table slowly backed out of the machine.

None of the MRI technicians said anything to me. I just hate that! Can't they tell a person if something's wrong, or at least let you know that everything is fine just to put you at ease? The "doctor" is always the only one who can give you the results.

"Listen, people," I wanted to say, "a photo shoot was just taken of *my* insides! Don't I have a *say* in this?" However, being the polite and timid person that I am, I lifted myself off the table without saying anything except "Thank you very much."

"They'll fax the results to your doctor," she said as I walked out of the room.

My head turned slightly towards the monitors, which clearly had my pictures plastered all over them. I glanced at the technicians, who were standing in front of them, and they were smiling. In fact, if I didn't know any better, I would have thought they were deliberately trying to block my view as I passed by.

"Maybe they don't want me to see the big mass sitting in the middle of my body," I thought.

I looked for some kind of reaction from one of them ... *anything*. Throw me a bone, will you? I quickly tried to analyze their behavior.

Well, they were laughing. That should be a good sign, right? Then again, maybe they were laughing to throw me off so I wouldn't worry until the doctor called to give me the bad news! It's amazing how much I can read into a situation within seconds and be way off track. All of this crossed my mind while I tippy-toed past each of them and even managed to flash a smile their way.

We went home and waited for Dr. Derini to call with the results. As soon as I walked in, I ran to see if there were any messages ... none yet. I sat down at the desk in my bedroom and stared at the phone.

"Please ring. Please ring. Please ring."

Rrrring!

The phone shuddered on my desk as the sound echoed through the house—like a Saturday morning *Bugs Bunny* cartoon, with his old-fashioned rotary phone flying in the air in anticipation of an extremely important phone call. The receiver shook with every sound, and I could see the words *Rrrring! Rrrring! Rrrring!* floating in a cloud above the phone.

In spite of all the waiting and anticipation, I allowed it to ring several times; in fact, I considered not answering it at all. I didn't want to get the bad news. I thought that maybe my answering machine could take it better than I could. After much self-debate, I finally reached over and picked up the receiver. It wasn't yet up to my ear as I spoke.

"Hello?"

"Hey, Mare. It's me."

It was my friend Maureen calling. I got off the phone quickly because I didn't want to tie up the line. The phone didn't ring again, but I had to leave for another test. I needed to have a bone scan to make sure the cancer hadn't spread to my bones.

Later the same day, my parents, Peter, and I went to a different office for a bone scan. As I lay on another table, the technicians injected me with a second contrast dye and rolled me back and forth on a huge, scary machine. When the test was over and I got up from the bed, one of the technicians, who was very nice, came over with a copy of the slides.

"I just wanted to let you know that everything is clear on your scan," he said with a big smile.

"Thank you! Thank you *so much!*"

I walked into the waiting room and looked at the crowd. The room was packed; many people were standing because there weren't enough seats. A few were holding bottles, which were filled with different colored liquids, and taking small, disgusted sips from them; others were waiting with worried and restless expressions.

I looked across the room and spotted my mom, my dad, and Peter. As their eyes met mine, the four of us walked towards each other and met in the center. The room seemed to quiet down and everyone's voice was reduced to whispers. A few eyes popped up from magazines and newspapers, and a few conversations stopped, while they turned to look at us.

My voice choked as I looked at my parents and at Peter.

"The scans are clear. Everything's fine."

The four of us hugged right there in the middle of the waiting room.

After we left, I called Dr. Derini's office because we still hadn't heard anything about the body scan from earlier in the day. Dawn answered the phone and told me that everything was clear on that scan, too! Once again, the four of us threw our arms around each and breathed collective sighs of relief.

Later that night, my sister Theresa and brother-in-law Mike came over. They had been on vacation and hadn't seen me since I found out about the cancer. My mom, sisters Margaret and Theresa, and I went up to my bedroom. I sat on the floor, fumbling through some things and trying to distract myself, and they all sat on my bed. Mom and Margaret updated Theresa on everything that had transpired during the week.

Theresa got up in the middle of the conversation and left the room; my mom quickly followed her. Margaret stayed behind, trying to make light conversation to divert my attention, but I just looked at the floor.

Growing up, we had arguments as any normal family does and, as you can imagine, we loved and adored each other just the same. We were always a tightly knit family. We carried on about silly things and, on occasion, chased after each other around the house. Nevertheless, and most importantly, we watched over and protected one another.

My brother and sisters were my role models when I was young—although, at the time, I would never ever admit that to them! When you're little, you *never* divulge information like that to a brother or sister because it can leave you in a very vulnerable position. Letting them know that I put them high on a pedestal and thought the world of them would leave me too exposed and defenseless during a good argument!

In addition to my siblings, my parents were trying to protect me. As helpless as they appeared to be, they were now on top of me with every step or breath I took. If I dropped something, they'd come running over to see if I were okay.

Were they uptight and high strung? Surely, they had every reason to be. Were they waiting for me to panic or explode? God knows I was about to do just that. Were they making sure that I didn't break? After all, I was being bent so far backwards, I just might snap!

Dr. Derini called me from Florida. He was away again—this time on vacation—and wanted to check in on me. He called as I was sitting on the couch in my pajamas, watching TV.

Naturally, I was wearing my pajamas. After all, sick people wear pajamas all the time, right? Once I was told that I had cancer, I didn't get dressed very often for the first couple of weeks. Pajamas, robe, and slippers were my everyday get-up.

I asked Dr. Derini a few questions, looking for some sort of encouragement. He told me that he probably got "most of it" and not to worry because he'd take good care of me.

Most of it? What's *that* supposed to mean? Is he kidding? There could be hundreds of cancer cells lurking in my body right now! That's like saying 100 murderers were set free, but *most* of them were captured. Either you got all of them, buddy, or you didn't. There are no in-betweens. Rationalizing doesn't work that way—at least not in the *Stolfa Book of Worries*.

After a long conversation, I finally hung up the phone feeling a little more confident—or at least I *think* I felt a little more confident.

"Let me go get my robe and slippers," I thought.

In fear of dying, I paced around the house. It wasn't just the thought of losing my life that tormented me. It was also the thought of losing all the people whom I loved so much. I couldn't bear the thought of not being with them anymore. I believe in God and in heaven, but I wasn't ready to go—not now. There were so many things that I still wanted to do.

I thought about how I would never get the chance to be married, have kids, and live the rest of my life. I felt robbed. I was looking forward to a bright future; to all the dreams, hopes, and promises that life has to offer. Who thought that life would offer me *cancer*?

Friends and family called to offer their love and support. They told me repeatedly how much courage they thought I had, but I had my own thoughts.

"A courageous person usually volunteers, doesn't she? She signs up. She's not drafted, right? She isn't thrown into a ring without boxing gloves where her rival is thrown at her, leaving her to swing her fists in the air fighting for her life, is she?"

"I don't think I can do this. I can't … I just can't," I said to my friend Lisa.

"Well, Mary, you have no choice. You *have* to fight."

Lisa was right: I had no choice. I would have to fight a battle I didn't ask for. I was an untrained soldier, standing in the front lines, forced to fight to the end against a faceless, malevolent enemy that had no rules or mercy. One of us would have to die, and I was terrified that it would be me.

I knew what I needed to do.

With tears pouring down my face, I started to pack for my journey—a journey I never would have chosen for myself. This would be the year I'd walk to hell and back.

One by one, I thought about how to place each piece into a small suitcase.

The first thing I packed was Faith. I folded it up and tucked it neatly inside.

Beside Faith, I placed Courage.

Then, I took Strength and set it next to both of them.

Next, I slowly picked up Hope, lifted it in front of my face, and gazed at it for a minute. I needed Hope to protect me from all of the fear and doubt that I knew would come my way. I tied a string to it and gently placed it around my neck.

I checked to make sure that I had all the Love ever given to me. Certainly I would need Love to help me find my way.

I was now ready to leave for my trip.

I've always felt as though everything in life happens for a reason. I believe events that transpire, both trials and triumphs, serve a purpose, and the people who cross our paths build our character, and shape and mold us into the people who we become.

I looked back on my life and wondered why cancer touched my history, beginning with my grandparents, and why I got it now. At 27 years old, I always imagined being married to Mr. Wonderful and starting a family. I'd have a great career and an active social life. The entire world would be at my fingertips. There would be so much fun and excitement in my future.

My mom always told me that I truly knew how to enjoy life. When she said it, I was living my life to the fullest. Being close to my family, having so many great friends, and dating always led me to many exciting new adventures and opportunities.

I pictured myself living my life, not fighting for it. Although everyone told me how much strength they thought I had, they failed to realize that it was they—not me—who held that strength. They were my strength because I didn't feel strong at the time. I felt as if I were falling into a bottomless pit.

Coming to my rescue, I saw the arms of every person who ever touched my life reaching out to catch me. I had a wonderful support system. Calls, cards, baskets, religious medals, gifts—especially angels—came to send me good wishes and blessings. People whom I didn't even know, who knew me through others, called and asked prayer groups to pray around the world for me.

As one friend said, "Well, Mary, that's the life you've built around you. The people surrounding you are the people you've chosen to share your life with."

Lisa said, "My friend, you are breaking hearts."

However, *my* heart broke every time I told one of these people that I was sick. I knew how everyone expected me to rise to the occasion and throw this disease back from where it came, never to return, but all that this scared little girl wanted to do was to crawl into a ball in the corner of a room somewhere and cry until it all went away.

It was incredible to see so many people come together. It was also incredible that I could have so many people around me and still feel so alone. Despite all of the love and support, I knew that ultimately it would have to be me, by myself, to either surrender or fight like hell to get my life back.

Throughout the day, I tried my best not to show fear. I saved my worst thoughts for the night when I was by myself—well, "by myself" for the most part; my parents could not get close enough to me.

One night, they literally pulled me into their bed and placed me between them. We watched TV, huddled under the covers. It was a tight squeeze with three adults, but they weren't about to let me leave. After a while, it was late and time to go to sleep. I kissed them goodnight and inched off the bed.

I crawled into my own bed and pulled the covers over my head. I shivered and cried, and clenched the old, yellow rosary beads I had since I was four years old. I buried my face into the pillow and wailed. I had to muffle my sobs so my mom and dad wouldn't hear. I continued to flip the pillow over as it became drenched in tears. Eventually, I fell asleep from exhaustion.

The next day, I thought about Dr. Mazza, who told me back in September that nothing was wrong. I also thought about having cancer at 27 years old. How long had the cancer been there? How did it end up like this? Was I eating the wrong foods all these years? Was it something I did—or didn't do—that caused it? Was I not a good enough person? Was I not exercising enough? How could this possibly happen?

I never allowed myself to ask, "Why me?" I always thought that asking God something like "Why me?" was like asking Him, "Why not someone else *instead* of me?" and cancer wasn't something I wished for anyone.

The next morning, I spoke to my friend Kate again. This conversation was much different than the last one. There were no jokes about tumors with eyeballs and teeth.

"You *will* beat this and be here to see Sean on his 25th birthday," referring to her one-year-old son.

Kate, along with her husband Steve and many other very good friends of mine, continued to visit or take me out to get my mind—or rather *try* to get my mind—off everything. However, no matter what I was doing, whom I was talking to, or where I went, the very same thought went through my mind: cancer.

I was in a diner with some friends, who were talking, laughing, and saying anything and everything other than the "Big C" word; however, the subject was clearly on *my* mind.

One of them asked me, "What are you going to have to eat?"

I thought, "Who, me? Well, I'm having cancer ... and you?"

They continued talking.

"Wasn't it funny last month when all of us...."

I continued thinking, "No, wait! You know what was even funnier? It was when I joked about having a cancerous tumor, and now I really *have* one!"

I sat there, listening to them laugh and talk, and joined in to make them think they were actually taking my mind off of—well, you know—cancer.

As doctors' visits, consultations, and tests continued, everyone went out of their way to keep me occupied because they didn't want me to have too much time to dwell on my illness. Although they tried very hard to keep my mind off cancer, it was apparently still on *their* minds.

I went to lunch with my friend Robin. While sitting at the table, I told her that I had thought about canceling our lunch date.

"I'm not feeling very well, Robin, and wasn't sure if I was up to going out."

She looked up from the menu, shrugged her shoulders, and simply said, "Mary, it wouldn't have been a big deal. Why didn't you just *cancer*?"

Her eyes widened as she bit down on her lip. We both looked at each other and burst out laughing.

For friends who lived too far away to scoop me up and take me out, there were alternative ways to keep me occupied.

My friend Suzanne now lives in California. Although our April Fools' Day prank never made it very far the day Grammy Rizzuto died—April 1, 1984— our friendship did.

Over the years, Suzanne and I dressed up and made home movies. We were always digging our hands into the cookie jar; that is, if we weren't trying to figure out a way to "sell" the cookie jar to make money! We attempted to start our own business—Magic and More—before we were 15, as well as other businesses, all of which never materialized, but our special bond lasted.

Despite being all grown up and working close to 100 hours a week, Suzanne threw on different costumes and filmed a home movie just for me. She publicly humiliated herself and her boyfriend at the time, and even included coupons that I could cash in if I wanted to see more of any one of the movie's characters.

Not long after receiving my home movie in the mail, I received a phone call from a coworker, who told me that the office took up a collection for a wig. They'd also made a donation to a breast cancer foundation in my name, and many of them participated in a cancer walk in honor of me.

We don't usually think about why we choose our friends. It goes back to the days in elementary school, standing on the ball field, when the gym teacher tells us to *pick a team*. We may not truly understand or comprehend the choices we make at that time, but it all comes together one day as we watch each and every one of our friends (our team) step up to the plate.

My friends Pam and Dan printed pins to wear at a cancer walk. Each one had my picture on it and said, "Walk for Mary."

I remember the moment that picture was taken. We were at a pub, which had over 800 different types of beers. We didn't try every one of them but came pretty close. At the end of the night, we were goofing around. I decided to grab things off the table and stuff them down my t-shirt: tablecloth, salt and pepper shakers, bottles, and whatever else was in front of me. As I was clowning around, one of my friends pointed the camera at me. I turned, put my arms up in the air, and smiled as the flash went off.

"Cheese!"

CHAPTER 8

Eeny, Meeny, Miny, Moe— Catch a Doctor by the Toe

Everyone told me to get a second opinion—"just in case." A friend of the family recommended Dr. Bogen, Chief of Breast Services at Memorial Sloan–Kettering Cancer Center in New York City. He had been interviewed on TV shows and was the subject of books and magazines about his accomplishments.

When my father originally called to get an appointment with Dr. Bogen, they said that they weren't able to fit me in right away; it would be months before the doctor could see me. My father thanked the woman on the phone and hung up. Moments later, he called back.

"Please fit my daughter in. She's only 27 years old," he pleaded.

They placed him on hold and, within minutes, I had an appointment for the following week. Since I felt bad telling my "angel" doctor that I was getting a second opinion, my dad let him know.

He also had another burning question for Dr. Derini. We had learned that an older woman, also named Mary, had a lumpectomy just before I did, and Dr. Derini also performed her surgery. Furthermore, she spelled her last name *exactly* like mine, except for one letter. Apparently, when we called to get my pathology report as well as other information for the "second opinion" doctor, we found out that her biopsy came back negative.

This is when my dad turned into Ben Stolfa, PI. He insisted that, since our names were almost identical, this woman could *really* be the one with cancer. Maybe somehow they accidentally switched our pathology reports. There was a mix-up, of course! Why didn't I think of that? Naturally, there's a "wild switcher" in the laboratory, who goes around swapping everyone's pathology reports, and I was the new victim! My father insisted that I wasn't the one with cancer and we have to let them know right away.

I was completely humiliated and begged him not to say anything to Dawn or Dr. Derini because he would sound crazy. I was too embarrassed to listen, and I walked out of the room when he called.

From the next room, I heard that they were indeed able to confirm my results: I had cancer and Mary Stolf-something-or-other did not. Even with this affirmation, Ben Stolfa, PI, would not let it go. He was determined to do more investigating.

The day finally came when my parents and I met with Dr. Bogen from Sloan. He nicely explained a disease about which we didn't understand or know and of which we were tremendously frightened. He clearly described all of the treatment options.

He reiterated everything that Dr. Derini had originally explained to us; however, I was still apprehensive, thinking that he might tell us something we hadn't already heard. I didn't want to know numbers, or whether he thought I had a good—or not so good—chance of living. As he continued talking, I clung to every word.

The three of us sat in front of his desk as he turned the computer monitor around to show us illustrations of the form of cancer he believed I had. He explained how the cancer must have broken out of the tumor and scattered throughout the entire region; however, his fancy three-dimensional pictures were a complete waste. My parents seemed distant, and I didn't see anything more than the haze that had formed over my eyes.

He explained how cancer cells were found inside of the milk ducts as well, which confirmed that the cancer originated in the breast and we weren't seeing another cancer that had metastasized.

"That's good," I thought. "Hadn't even thought of that one."

Next came a crash course on cancer, and we sat in disbelief. I wanted to jump out of my skin, but I watched as he pointed at the screen and showed us pictures of what was most likely in my chest. His calmness emanated throughout the room.

Despite his somber tone, and out of sheer anxiety, I still felt like rising out of my seat, clutching onto the walls, digging my fingernails into the paint, and climbing up to the ceiling to escape—one hand after another.

In my mind, suspended in the air by my fingernails, I imagined turning to Dr. Bogen and saying, "Go on, Doc. I'm listening. Please continue."

Dr. Bogen offered two options. They could do a lumpectomy and extract more tissue to see if the borders were clear of cancer and, if they were clear, not go any further. They could also do a modified radical mastectomy to remove my breast and a number of lymph nodes.

I had already made up my mind before I walked into his office that day.

I would have a mastectomy.

"I don't want this breast anymore," I thought. "I don't want anything to do with it. Just take it away. It disgusts me. I can't look at it or stand the thought of how it turned on me. It's repulsive and I need to get it off of my chest."

From the day I found out it was cancerous, I was barely able to look at my breast anymore. It felt as if I had a pack of explosives attached to me, which could explode at any given moment. I wanted it removed as quickly as possible.

I can't explain how it feels to give up a part of your body with which you've lived for your entire life. When I glanced at pictures that my mom had out or ones hanging on the walls around the house, I looked down at my chest. I thought about when those pictures were taken and didn't know what I would be losing in the future. What a huge loss it would be. I felt that losing half my chest was like losing half my womanhood.

The three of us didn't utter a word until my father cleared his throat. Dr. Bogen stopped talking and silence quickly filled the room. My dad looked him unswervingly in the eye.

"If it were your child, what would you do?"

Without hesitation, Dr. Bogen immediately responded that he would undoubtedly recommend a mastectomy. *There!* The decision was made and I agreed. He also recommended chemotherapy and radiation, which we would discuss later.

Then, Ben Stolfa, PI, talked to Dr. Bogen, Chief of Breast Services, about "The Case of the Jumbled Pathology Report." My dad asked Dr. Bogen what we could do to confirm that the biopsy slides weren't an accidental mix-up with the other woman named Mary.

My head dropped down—I might have even gasped—and I curled up in my seat with embarrassment as the words left my father's mouth. It's at these moments when you wish that life was a video where you can press stop, rewind, and then delete.

To my surprise, Dr. Bogen took him seriously. Without skipping a beat, Dr. Bogen offered to perform a fine needle biopsy, or I could just wait until the surgery to confirm that it was definitely cancer. He didn't recommend a mastectomy without knowing because that would mean that I would go into surgery uncertain of whether or not I had cancer and possibly wake up with one breast.

A few days after the consultation, I decided to have him aspirate my breast, and Peter and Kate took me back to Sloan to have it done. We stepped into the elevator along with a couple of other people and pressed the button. The doors closed and the elevator began to move.

"*Slam!*"

All of a sudden, the elevator stopped.

"What now?" I thought.

Kate and Peter simultaneously swung their heads around to look at me—claustrophobic me. My eyes popped out as I backed towards the elevator wall behind everyone. Very calmly—perhaps too calmly—one of the other passengers pressed the emergency button and a voice came out of the speaker.

"Hello? *Hello?*"

The passenger quietly whispered, "Yes. The elevator seems to be stuck. Can you help us?"

"Hello? Is anyone there? *Hello?*"

The man next to me asked faintly, "Yes. Can you *help* us? Apparently, the elevator has stopped."

Kate looked over at me again, trying to give me a reassuring smile, as the two other passengers were getting us nowhere fast. All I saw was Kate, wearing a warped, crooked, nervous smile—her failed attempt to make me feel better.

Peter wasn't doing much better. He was swinging his head all over the place: from the speaker, at me, back to the other passenger, at me again, at the speaker, at the man, around to me once more, and then over to Kate—round and round and back again to the speaker.

He had just about stopped to look over at me again when all hell broke loose. After the two strangers softly repeated themselves several times, Kate knew that I was just about to lose it, so she decided to push everyone out of the way and promptly walked up to the microphone.

Putting her face directly in front of the speaker, she shouted, "We're stuck! Help us! We need help! We're stuck in the elevator! Get us out of here!"

Minutes later, the elevator began to move.

"Not off to a great start today," I thought.

Dr. Bogen performed a biopsy and, by the next day, had confirmed the results to be positive; however, I still had to choose a plastic surgeon for the reconstruction. We consulted with a plastic surgeon from North Shore University Hospital on Long Island, whom I didn't particularly like.

Dr. Silver was a bit self-centered and arrogant. He pranced into the examination room with a flashy, pinstriped, expensive suit; gaudy jewelry; fake tan; whitened teeth; dyed and hair-sprayed hair whirled into a bouffant. He was scary-looking fake to me and had the personality to match. He probably looks in the mirror every day and says, "You're hot, man!" and gives himself a wink as he positions his hand like a gun and shoots.

"You are no longer going to have a breast," Dr. Silver said. "Do you understand that? The reconstruction will leave you with only a mound. Just a mound, that's all. You will never have a real breast there again," he insensitively repeated.

He had no bedside manner and overemphasized something he didn't have to overemphasize. I wasn't born yesterday. I knew it would be an implant in my chest and certainly didn't need this pompous ass rubbing it in my face. I think he could have used a little surgery on his ego.

Jesse, my new friend from the support group that Dr. Derini had me speak with, referred me to another plastic surgeon that I really liked. My mom and I left for the appointment to see Dr. Ziger. My dad had something to take care of beforehand, and he was going to catch up with us later. In the middle of the consultation, which was a very serious talk about my prospective options, we heard a knock at the door.

"*Hello?*" we heard from the hallway. "Anyone in there?" The banging and fumbling noises continued, and then we heard, "Do I have the right room?"

The door opened slowly and my dad's face appeared. As he entered, he kept knocking the door with the cane he used on occasion.

"Hey, how ya doin'?" he asked, stumbling towards the doctor to shake his hand.

Everyone sat there watching as my dad looked around for a minute or two, deciding where to sit. He settled down between my mom and me, and found the right place for his cane so it wouldn't fall.

Dr. Ziger continued the conversation—a conversation that was going well *before* my dad got there.

"Anyway," the doctor continued, "as I was saying, I can certainly give you as close as possible to what a natural breast would look like."

As the good doctor explained this, my father suddenly chose to interrupt.

"Um … let me ask you a question."

Simultaneously, my mom and I swung our heads around to look at my father.

"Oh, no, not a question," I thought. "Please not a question." If I could have stretched out my arms and covered his mouth, I would have. I wanted to scream to the high heavens, "Nooooooo! Pul-ease, Dad, don't *do* it!"

I couldn't stop him, so I just sat there. I squeezed my hands together and curled up my toes inside of my sneakers. I took a quick glimpse at my mother and saw that she was wearing her fake smile—the one she wears when she is nervous and embarrassed but clearly trying to be polite. This time, though, it was worse: Inquisitive eyebrows went up as her head tilted to one side. I knew it was bad when her eyebrows rose.

She was just as terrified as I was, and even the doctor was almost on the edge of his seat, waiting to see what was going to happen next. He looked back and forth at my mom, my dad, and me, and things quickly turned from bad to worse.

"It can't be *that* bad, could it?" I thought.

I'm sure the doctor was thinking the same thing. He'd probably been asked a million questions and interrogated about anything and everything imaginable.

Well, I guess not *everything*.

With one long breath, my dad looked the doctor straight in the eye and asked, "Is there any way that I can donate my nipple to my daughter? I'd give her anything in the world, so if there's any way you can give it to her, then I want her to have it."

He sat up straight and patted his chest.

My mom's face froze with her fake smile. I laid my elbow on the arm of the chair and threw my hand over my face. I tried not to look at Dr. Ziger, but I couldn't help myself. I peeked out from between my fingers. I guess "astonished" would be an appropriate description for his look. I couldn't bear to see anymore, so I quickly buried my face back into my hand.

The room was completely silent. No one made a move or uttered a word for several minutes. After an extremely uncomfortable and lengthy pause, which seemed to last for hours, the cordial plastic surgeon swallowed hard, and then turned to my father.

"Mr. Stolfa, I would have won the Nobel Prize if I were able to do something like that."

"Oh? Okay," my father responded, seemingly surprised, as if he were thinking, "If they can transplant a heart, what would be difficult about a tiny nipple?" He turned to the doctor and said, "Well, I just figured I'd ask."

At this point in my life, everybody wanted to donate something to me. My sister Margaret wanted to give me her thick hair for a wig if mine fell out during chemotherapy, my sister Theresa offered me her "eggs" if I became infertile from the chemo, and now my dad wanted to give me his nipple!

By the end of the week, I was tired of meeting doctors and hearing about all the horrible things that I needed to do. Like it or not, we had an appointment with another plastic surgeon from Sloan, who worked with Dr. Bogen on a regular basis.

My mother, my father, and I walked into Dr. Dia's office and checked in. The waiting room clearly displayed the effects of cancer, and the patients were as I hopeful as I that the doctor would make them look like they did before cancer changed them. I kept my head down and the three of us took our seats.

My mom talked to me, and my dad cracked jokes, both trying to keep me calm; however, my eyes darted all over the place because I didn't want to look at the person directly in front of me. I also didn't want to look at the person beside me, diagonally across, or anywhere else.

I stared at the dots on the floor and became fixated on them. After some time had passed, though, I couldn't do it any longer, so I looked up and took a quick glimpse at some of the people surrounding us.

A woman, who sat diagonally across from me, was missing one of her eyes—one eye was wide open and the other lid was sewn shut. Beside her sat a man with one of his ears missing. It looked as if a large piece of skin, taken from another part of his body, covered the area where his ear must have been. I looked across the room and saw another man in a wheelchair with one of his legs missing.

It was heart wrenching. I felt as though I walked onto the set of a dreadful horror movie. It was so painful to see what cancer had done to these innocent people, and my heart broke for all of them. Trying to make sense of it all, I sat there for the next three hours, my clammy hands twisting and squeezing in fear.

Can a person ever make sense of it all? Is there any meaning or reason to justify something so cruel and unkind? I couldn't see any fairness about being left with one eye, one ear, or one leg. No one deserves that.

I sank into my chair and continued to think about life and the reason why things happen. I prayed for this room full of people and was sad for each one of them. As I glanced around the room, I had an epiphany. Somehow, it all seemed to be an enormous lesson. I realized that my situation—having to trade one breast in exchange for my life—wasn't as bad as I thought it was.

From that moment, I vowed never to complain about what I was losing. Instead, I would focus on what I was gaining: *my life.* I also realized that I wasn't losing my womanhood.

That day, I came to terms with what was happening to me and learned a significant and valuable lesson. It's amazing how a room full of strangers can teach you something so priceless. Without a word, every one of those courageous people had shown me that this was a victory and not a defeat in my life. I was winning much more than the breast I was losing.

After meeting with Dr. Dia, my mother, my father, and I walked out of the office and into the hallway. My father pressed the button, and we waited for the elevator. Shortly thereafter, a young man walked up beside me and waited along with us. I noticed that his hair was shaved, but I didn't think much of it. He didn't look like a patient to me.

I had been observing everyone who walked the halls of the hospital each time I went, wondering about them: Were they cancer patients? What type of cancer did they have? How long have they had it?

For a moment, I thought that this young man might have been visiting someone in the hospital, but I didn't give much thought to it. I concluded that he was just a visitor, and then glanced towards the elevator.

I looked back over at him and he seemed impatient. His eyes flitted as if he were nervous and didn't know where or what to focus on. As he slowly turned to the side, I realized why he was there. A swollen red scar ran across the other side of his head. It was sunken and looked like part of his skull was missing. My God! Brain cancer! Tears came to my eyes as the elevator doors opened and we all stepped in.

After meeting with two breast surgeons and three plastic surgeons, I had to make some decisions. My parents left the choices up to me because I was the one who needed to decide where I would get treatment. They didn't give me their opinion but instead said that they would take me to the ends of the earth—all the way into New York City to Sloan-Kettering or just a few miles away on Long Island to North Shore University Hospital.

I was determined to get well and live out the rest of my life. Both hospitals and doctors were wonderful, but I decided to go with Dr. Bogen as my breast surgeon and Dr. Dia as my plastic surgeon, who were both at Sloan-Kettering.

The mastectomy was scheduled for April 3rd.

I was trying to make the right decisions with everything thrown at me all at once: the hospital, the doctor, the surgery, the treatment, and fertilization. My mind was all over the place, and I began to think a bit illogically about other areas of my life.

I called my friend Jennifer and told her that I thought I should break up with Peter. I was unsure if I'd ever be able to have kids and didn't want to make him stay. I didn't know what my future held or if I even *had* a future. I needed to do the right thing and let him go.

Minutes later, I received a call from Peter, asking me what was going on.

"Well, I just wanted to spare you, Peter. I want to handle this with integrity and dignity. I don't want you to get hurt."

"Don't worry about me," he said.

He explained how much he loved me and how there was no turning back now. He told me that we needed to focus on what was in front of us and on my health. He insisted that we would do it *together*. It was hard keeping a positive outlook when it seemed that our world was crashing down before our eyes but, with each new uncertainty, we grew closer. We encountered more during our short-lived dating period than most people do in a 50-year marriage.

My sister Margaret and I are three years apart and share the same birthday—March 23rd—and my family got together as usual to celebrate. In addition to my brother Nicholas and my sister Theresa, I've always looked up to Margaret.

Growing up, I was the tough tomboy and Margaret was the petite princess. I wanted to be just like her when I was little; maybe that's why I used to wear her clothes all the time. It's nice for her to hear that now, but she never appreciated it when I was 16 years old, walking out the front door and wearing her favorite shirt.

We'd always fuss about having the same birthday and argue over who stole whose birthday. She'd claim how she was here first, and I'd fight about how she took it from me three years before I got the chance. Over the years, we'd pretend how we didn't like sharing the same day, but we always knew how special it really was. We'd never admit it, but we actually loved the fact that we shared the same day.

Ten days before my mastectomy, this birthday would be different. It meant more than the other ones because this year it was a celebration of life.

The room was completely silent as everyone looked at Margaret and me. We reached towards the candles on our birthday cakes and took deep breaths. We closed our eyes and exhaled as we made a shared wish.

The flame went out and, as smoke slowly rose from the candles, we looked at each other. For the first time in 28 years, we knew exactly what the other one had wished for.

CHAPTER 9

"Dear Cancer, I Need to Get Something off My Chest."

woke up on the morning of April 3rd with a knot in my stomach. I forced myself to get up, get dressed, and leave the house. My father, my mother, and I did not say much during the car ride. Sadly, taking one step at a time, I walked into the hospital to have my mastectomy. Completely overwhelmed with feelings of grief and devastation, at 28 years old and in the prime of my life, the surgeon would cut off my breast this morning.

Shortly after I arrived, the nurses walked me into the changing room to put on my gown and robe. As I took off my clothes, one piece at a time, I placed them into a plastic bag. Before I put on the gown, I slowly looked at the mirror in front of me. This would be the last time I would ever see myself like this.

My eyes began to water, my bottom lip quivered, my head dropped down, and I literally felt my heart sink deeply inside my chest. I picked up the gown, opened it, and inserted my arms. I put on the hospitals socks and then slipped a Blessed Mother medal, which my friend Kerri had given me, down into the sock.

I tucked my hair into a paper hat, clenched my old yellow rosary beads, and then walked back to the waiting room to sit down with the rest of my family. After a while, the nurse still hadn't called me in, so I began to get restless. I took out my cell phone and made a few calls to some other family members and friends.

At the pre-op appointment, the hospital staff had asked me if I wanted a nun to pray with me before the mastectomy. My mom jumped at the chance and said yes. Before long, a nun walked into the waiting room and looked directly at me.

"Mary?"

"Yes, I'm Mary."

"I came to say a prayer with you."

The nun took my hand, and everyone joined in and prayed. My mom immediately started to cry. After we finished and the nun walked away, I turned to my mother and smirked in an unsuccessful attempt to make her laugh.

"Oh, will you just get *over* it already!"

Not long after that, the doctors were finally ready and one of the nurses came to escort me. With my Blessed Mother medal stuffed into my sock, and my rosary beads in my hand, I swallowed hard as I hugged and kissed my family and friends good-bye.

I wasn't scared of the surgery, of being put to sleep, or of them cutting me. I was scared of what I was going to see after I woke up. I was completely heartbroken. To reassure everyone, I put on a fake smile, which I was barely able to muster, and then walked arm and arm with the nurse through the double steel doors and into the operating room.

I stopped and looked at the room. There were beeping, suctioning, pumping, and clicking sounds all around me, and a team of doctors and nurses prepared for the mastectomy. There was an almost indescribable scent—a sickly, disinfected, sanitized kind of smell that I'll never forget—permeating the room, like alcohol and laughing gas from the dentist's office. The room was cold and the fluorescent lights glared off the stainless steel table in the center of the room. Everyone wore masks.

As we walked, the nurse squeezed my hand.

"Are you okay?"

I nodded while examining all the sophisticated computers, machines, tubes, and equipment around me. My legs were weak and shaky, so I concentrated on putting one foot in front of the other as she walked me over to the operating table. I lay on the cold, steel table, shivering and trying to keep from crying.

She placed a blanket over me and slipped off my gown. I was completely naked with just the blanket draped across me. I clenched my teeth to stop them from chattering, and then clasped both my hands to stop them from shaking.

One of the other nurses grabbed my hands and told me that everything was going to be okay. As nurses began hooking me up to a few of the fancy machines, I glanced over at the double steel doors and saw Dr. Bogen enter.

"It's okay," the nurse kept saying as she held my hands.

The anesthesiologist placed a large mask over my face and told me to take deep breaths. I couldn't hold back anymore and tears welled up as my eyes slowly closed.

I woke up in the recovery room and realized that my mom was holding my hand. I squeezed her hand tightly with what little strength I had.

"Please, don't let me go," I thought, and I meant it in every sense.

When I first found out that I had cancer, my mom told me that she knew I loved life too much to give up … and I did. What frightened me the most was that the choice would not be mine to make.

As the anesthesia wore off, the hospital staff gave me several other medications; for the most part, I was still incoherent. One by one, everybody came to see me, but my eyes were still very blurry. As my vision slowly began to clear up, I saw a hazy figure leaning over the bed to kiss me. It was my dad. He looked at me with a reassuring look and then smiled, as if to tell me that everything was going to be okay.

I felt like a baby once again, falling flat on my face and looking for my parents to help me back up … to help me stand … to help me be strong again. I knew that my mom and dad wouldn't let go of me unless they were absolutely sure I was able to stand on my own.

Damn this cancer. *Damn* it for putting me in this hospital and feeling doubtful about my future. *Damn* it for making my parents have to teach me again about all the valuable lessons of what life is really about—that, in fact, it is a beautiful miracle and you can't let doubt or fear overcome how good life can really be. During these past few weeks, I was beginning to forget.

After my father backed away from the bed, I saw a policeman coming towards me. It was Peter! With a nervous, forced smile, he gave me a gentle kiss on my forehead. My friend Christine also came in and held my hand for a while. Then Ann Marie, other friends, and family members entered, one by one.

All of a sudden, I felt my heart beginning to pound. It was violently beating and I felt as if it would burst through my chest at any moment. *Boom! Boom! Boom!* I thought I was having a heart attack.

The monitors started to make very loud and rapid beeping sounds. I couldn't move, but I watched as everyone backed away from my bed. A group of nurses and doctors ran towards me from every direction and determined that I was having an allergic reaction to one of the medications.

At some point during the commotion, one of the doctors injected something into my IV line. A few seconds later, my heart settled down and the panic was over. All of this happened within seconds, but it seemed like hours.

Not long after that, the nurse wheeled me to my room where the rest of my family and friends were waiting. They pushed my bed against the wall and locked it, and then pulled down the side railing.

The morphine began to wear off; however, I decided that I didn't want any more painkillers—other than Tylenol—because of the reaction I had suffered in the recovery room. *Stupid, stupid patient.*

It got late. Peter finally went home, but my mom wouldn't leave my side. She slept on a chair at the foot of my bed.

I was awake the entire night, just lying there and staring at the ceiling, barely able to move an inch. If I had to reposition myself—even the tiniest bit—I would cry out in pain. They wrapped layers of gauze, bandages, tape, and elastic around me. Underneath it all, it felt as if they had scraped out the entire left side of my chest with a dull carving knife. It even hurt to breathe, so I took small, shallow breaths. I was in agonizing pain but refused even an aspirin.

Everything had quieted down until a rush of nurses suddenly burst into the room. They quickly closed the curtain in the middle, and I could hear several people coming in and out on the other side. Then I saw a woman wheeled in on a gurney.

From the moment Thelma entered the room, she was moaning and crying out in horrific pain. I'll never forget the fear in her voice when she asked the doctor if she was "going to die."

The next day, Thelma was screaming in pain again. After we called the nurse to get her pain medication, I was very upset to hear someone in that much agony. It was heart wrenching. I lay in my bed and cried for her. I stared at the TV as tears poured down my face.

One of the nurses came in to clean out my drains, which they had sewn into my side to release any excess fluid that might build up in my chest. The nurse bent down on the floor next to me. As she was cleaning the drains, she looked right at me.

"You know that has nothing to do with you, right?" She nodded towards the curtain that separated me from Thelma. "She has a different type of cancer, and her circumstances are completely different."

I lifted my hand to wipe my eyes and nose.

"I know, but I still feel bad for her."

Later that day, they switched me to another room. With my left arm locked into place on one side, I wheeled my IV pole down the hall with my right hand and checked on Thelma. A family member told me that she was doing a little better.

My mom stayed with me again that night. I was still in too much pain to sleep. I lay in bed awake. Even a minor attempt at repositioning caused horrific pain. The room was quiet. You could hear a pin drop; that is, until the lion was unleashed.

Let me tell you that, when my mother falls asleep, *she falls asleep*. She snores like a roaring lion … and not just *any* lion. She snores like the Queen of the Jungle!

"*Roooooar!*"

My mom began snoring, drooling, gurgling, and making any and every other kind of sound imaginable.

"Mom," I whispered.

No response.

"*Mom!*" I said a little louder.

I wanted to wake *her* up, not my roommate, unless she was already awake from Leona the Lion.

My mom wasn't budging.

I looked over at the nightstand and spotted a role of bandaging tape. I slowly lifted up my good arm and grabbed it. Aiming at her backside, I swung the tape at my poor mother in the hopes of somehow getting her attention.

Bang! I missed and the tape hit the chair.

I searched the nightstand for another tossable object. I grabbed a small pill cup and chucked it across the room. I finally managed to hit her, but unfortunately the blow wasn't hard enough to wake Sleeping Beauty.

Now I had to get tough.

I looked over at my IV pole. Well, now, *that's* an idea! With my other hand, I grabbed it and, with one hard swoop, pushed it in the direction of her chair.

Dammit! Not far enough.

I carefully pulled the pole back towards me by using the tubing from the line. With all the strength my weak body was able to pull together, I once again swung the pole in her direction and watched it roll straight for her chair.

"Go! Go! Go!" I thought.

The IV bag swung back as the pole glided across the shiny, waxed floor. I watched the long tube, which ran from the needle in my arm up to the IV bag, hanging from the pole. It dangled loosely onto the floor but slowly began to rise into the air and tighten as it made its way to my mother.

Slam ... I hit her!

With one loud snort, she lifted her head up ever so slightly.

"Mom, you're snoring *so loud!*"

"Oh, oh. Okay, okay," she said as she lay her head back down.

Two minutes later, it started all over again. I dropped my head on my pillow. If I had a white flag somewhere under my blanket, I would have waved it in the air. I surrender!

During the day, the nurses came in on a regular basis to empty my drains. They also had to teach me how to do it since the drains would remain for the next two weeks after I went home.

Every time they cleaned the drains, they'd ask, "Did you look yet?"

"Did I look?" I thought. "Did I look at my deformed body?"

"No, not yet," I told them.

It hadn't even been 24 hours and they wanted me to look.

When one of the nurses came in to change my bandages, she sat down on my bed. She put on rubber gloves and placed the alcohol swabs, tape, and fresh gauze beside us. I slowly unsnapped my gown by my shoulder and lowered my sleeve.

As she peeled back the bandages, she looked up at me and softly said, "Why don't you take a look?"

I did but not at my chest. I rolled my eyes to the side and looked towards the floor instead ... but she thought I had looked. I would when I was ready, but what was the sense of rushing it? My breast wasn't there now, and it still wouldn't be there later.

Although I had reconstructive surgery, it was incomplete. They inserted a "tissue expander" underneath the muscle in my chest, with a port underneath the skin. They would inject this port on a weekly basis with saline to increase the size and stretch out the skin slowly. Eventually they would replace this tissue expander with a permanent implant. For now, it had very little saline in it and was still very flat—at least from what I could see with my hospital gown over me.

At one point, I went to the bathroom and took off the elastic wrapped around me. I peeled the bandages back with my left hand and, without looking, placed my right hand over the mastectomy. It felt warm, and I felt the rough string from the stitches.

I covered the entire area with my right hand and slowly looked down. Dark, black stitches protruded between each of my five fingers. I couldn't muster the courage to move my hand away, so I lifted my head up and pulled the gauze over my chest.

I quietly sat down on the toilet seat and began to cry.

I made it through the night but, by morning, I wanted out! I was scared and wanted to be safe at home again. I begged my friends and family, who came to visit, to take me with them, but nobody would budge. I pleaded with everyone, but they all gave me the same pitiful look, put their heads down, and sighed.

"I'm sorry, but I just can't."

When Kate came to visit, she helped me to the bathroom and I started pleading with her.

"Please, I just want to go *home*, Kate. All of these sick people are scaring me. Please take me home."

I didn't realize that I was one of those sick people, too; however, I *did* realize that, if I wanted to escape, I would have to do it on my own, even if it meant getting on my hands and knees, begging for a discharge.

Peter stayed with me that night. After another restless night, I was up at the crack of dawn. The doctors did their rounds at 7:30 each morning. The following morning, I was up by 6:30, getting myself ready. I felt like a truck had run over me but, no matter what, come hell or high water, I was going home!

I washed, brushed my hair and teeth, and gently put on a clean hospital gown. Even though I was barely able to lift my arm, I actually put on make-up. I propped myself up in a chair, faced it directly in front of the door, and waited for the doctors to come to my room: the "Patients Who Are Miraculously All Better After Only One Day" room.

Two doctors—part of Dr. Dia's team—walked in. I managed a phony smile as beads of sweat formed on my forehead. With my right hand, I lowered my gown to show them my war scar.

"How do you feel?" they asked, while inspecting my wound.

"Good! I'm feeling good!"

I lied. If there were ever an Academy Award performance given at Memorial Sloan–Kettering, it was in my room that morning. Believing me, and without hesitation, the doctors discharged me. I was finally going home!

Peter drove very carefully, but even the smallest potholes jolted the car, sending a wrenching pain through my chest. Each time the car dipped into a hole, turned, or even changed lanes, our faces would cringe.

When I first walked through the front door, I headed straight for my bedroom. I walked in to see a huge, brand new color TV that Theresa and Mike had bought for me. My eyes lit up and I smiled as I sat down on my bed.

"I cannot *believe* they did this for me!"

As I looked around at my pictures, trinkets, and memorabilia, I began to think. It took 28 long years to build my life into what it was, and only 28 short seconds to be told that I had cancer and have it all shattered into a thousand pieces. I didn't know where or how to even begin to put my life back together.

I sat there for a very long time. Everything happened so fast. Making decision after decision about doctors, surgeries, and treatments, now I was sitting where it all started—in my bedroom—and I had a huge cut running across my chest.

It all came to this.

Gradually, I stood up from my bed and walked over to the dresser. It was time to empty out my drains. As I stood in front of the mirror, I lifted up my shirt and carefully took it off. I still couldn't move my left arm, so I wrapped the sleeve around my elbow and pulled it off from underneath. My shirt fell to the floor.

I delicately peeled back the tape, and then lifted the gauze from my chest. I placed the bandage on the dresser. I closed my eyes, raised my head, and then reluctantly looked at the mirror.

I looked.

I finally looked.

I stood there, staring at my chest through the mirror. My lungs filled with air as I gasped and then let out a cry under my breath.

"*O-h, m-y G-o-d.*"

As I stood there, unable to mutter a word, my eyes welled up with tears and my head slumped down in despair from what was looking back at me. I stared at the dark stitches that ran across my bare chest. I slowly turned to the side and saw tubes, which led to drains, protruding from my armpit. They had sewn them into my side.

It looked like a scene from the movie *Frankenstein*, and I was completely devastated. I inched over to my bed, emptied out my drains, and then crawled into bed.

The following week, I was back at Sloan for my post-op appointment with my parents. Dr. Bogen was going to examine the incision and tell me what further treatments, if any, I would need. We sat in the examining room, waiting for over an hour and a half.

After a grueling and agonizing wait, Dr. Bogen walked in. He sat directly in front of me, opened up a slim manila folder, and read the results from the mastectomy.

With one deep breath, I gathered all of the strength and courage I had and looked him straight in the eyes. I was face to face with the man who was going to tell me my future. I watched every move he made and focused on his every word.

He explained how there hadn't been any surprises.

"Surprises?" I thought. "What's that supposed to mean? Like a surprise when someone jumps out of a cake? I didn't know there could be a surprise. What kind?"

He meant that there was no more cancer than what they had originally anticipated; I didn't even realize there could have been. I thought the scans had already confirmed that fact. Thank God I didn't know *that* before the surgery.

Dr. Bogen continued by saying that I made the right choice to have the mastectomy because the cancer was in various places within my breast. There were 22 positive lymph nodes out of the 34 extracted. The cancer had gone to Level 3 nodes, which meant that the cancer had traveled fairly deeply inside of me.

"Pretty bad," I thought.

"The tissue in your left breast, where the tumor had been, was poorly differentiated, high grade, infiltrating carcinoma associated with extensive lymphovascular invasion. The cancer was most likely in the surrounding area, since several biopsies came back positive."

Then, as I sat on the examining table, my heart seemed to drop into my stomach. My throat began to close up and my body actually began to shake. My hands gripped onto one another as I squeezed and pulled at my fingers because, if I let them loose, every finger would have been trembling.

Dr. Bogen continued to say how the cancer had a "spray effect," meaning that there were traces of it all around the area. There were several swollen lymph nodes, cysts, and smaller tumors within the region. I would most likely need six months of chemotherapy followed by one month of radiation, but the chemotherapy wouldn't start for another six weeks since my body needed time to heal from the surgery.

Chemotherapy kills your immune system and radiation causes cancer, yet both fight cancer cells. Ironic, isn't it? Figure that one out.

"I can recommend an oncologist for you, if you'd like," he said. "Most of them are doom and gloom," he grinned and then winked at me, "but I'll get you a good one."

If I were eligible and agreed to participate, he offered, I may be able to participate in a clinical trial.

My nerves were doing back flips because I saw the walls shaking back and forth. Everything began to look distorted and I couldn't focus on any one thing. It was difficult to talk from the shock.

I looked at my parents. They just sat there stunned with their jaws hanging open. Not a peep came out of either one of them.

My voice shook as I finally got the courage to ask a question.

"Well, um … uh, Dr. Bogen?"

"Yes, Mary?"

"So, what um … uh, what do … um … what do you think my prognosis might be?" I asked, as my eyes welled up with tears.

That was the hardest question I have ever asked anyone in my entire life. I was asking him how long I had to live. I felt terror and fear shoot through my body like a bolt of lightning—from the top of my head to the tips of each of my toes. My world stopped for that one brief moment as I waited for his answer.

He leaned in towards me.

"Well, let me put it this way, Mary. I'll tell you a story. There was once a sick man whose doctor told him that he only had two years to live. Two years later, the doctor died, so the man went to another doctor. This new doctor told him the same thing—that he only had two years to live. After another two years, which was four years after the original doctor told him he was going to die, *that* doctor died. Then, he went to *another* doctor. This doctor was scared to tell him anything!"

He never gave me a straight answer. I don't think he wanted to tell me. I guess his point was that nobody can really tell you for sure how long you have to live.

I still wanted to crawl into a corner and shrivel up into the scared little girl I felt that I was. Somehow, I found the strength to lift up my chin from the floor and walk out of the hospital. I was becoming a stronger person because I had no other choice than to persevere.

Placing my fear aside, I needed to pick myself up with the strength and confidence of a first-place winner, not the defeat of a runner-up. No one comes in second or third place in the game of cancer. You win or you lose ... and I was going to win.

CHAPTER 10

Shall I Wear My Heart on My Sleeve or My Ovary in My Arm?

Despite my decision not to have Dr. Derini perform my mastectomy, Dawn, his nurse, continued to send me invitations to breast cancer seminars; I attended one of them a month or so after my surgery.

My friend Gayle, whom Dr. Derini was treating, was going to the seminar, and Lisa offered to drive me there. Lisa and I met up with Gayle and her husband Chris when we arrived.

Dawn spotted me immediately. She was behind a table in front of the main door but quickly jumped up to give me a big kiss and hug hello. She said that she had been a little worried because they sent me invitations but I never responded to any of them. I guess I just wasn't ready.

A few minutes later, I turned to the side and saw Dr. Derini. Being a kind person and professional doctor that I knew him to be, he walked towards me and gave me a huge hug that lasted for quite a while. After the seminar, I spoke with both of them. I told them about my surgery and the 22 positive lymph nodes.

Dawn turned to me and asked, "Are you scared?"

My head sank down as I muttered, "I'm fine. I know that everything is going to be okay."

I guess I felt that if I said it enough, I'd really believe it.

Over the next few weeks, as I was recovering from the surgery, my parents began their search for an oncologist. Although Dr. Bogen gave me the name of one, I wanted to explore my options. After getting recommendations from everyone about who was the best, who was the worst, who was nice, and who wasn't so nice, my parents and I found ourselves in the office of a doctor close to home.

We walked into a small, cramped office and the receptionist led us to the back. After Dr. Hern cleared off piles of paper from one of the chairs, we sat down in front of his desk. It was a dark, old wooden desk with stacks of papers scattered over the top.

Dr. Hern opened a folder containing paperwork, which I had filled out in the waiting room, and copies of my surgical and pathology reports, which the hospital had faxed to the office before I arrived. We discussed the standard course of chemotherapy for breast cancer, and he related that it would most likely be his suggested treatment for me.

As he glanced up from the paperwork through his half-glasses, he wore a surprised look.

"Wow! Twenty-two? I've never treated anyone with so many positive lymph nodes."

He harped on this particular fact for some time.

"Okay, okay!" I thought. "Is this supposed to make me feel better?" As I sat in front of him, shocked at what he was admitting, I thought, "... and you *still* will never have treated anyone with 22 positive lymph nodes!"

We thanked him for his time and left ... never *ever* to return.

When we got home, I set up an appointment with the oncologist from Sloan whom Dr. Bogen had recommended. Maybe *she'll* have treated someone with 22 positive lymph nodes?

I was also referred to a fertility clinic since there was a chance that chemo might leave me infertile. The appointment was for the following week with a specialist in New York. Both my mom and friend Jennifer planned to take me.

If anyone could make me laugh while on my way to a fertility clinic, it was Jennifer.

We were very late and stumbled into the fertility clinic. After arriving, I filled out some paperwork and saw the doctor right away. Shortly after our conversation began, "Dr. Frankenstein" suggested performing some new type of experimental surgery on me.

I would be the second patient to have one of my ovaries taken out and placed inside my arm. He told me that this would be a great alternative because I wouldn't have enough time before chemotherapy started to freeze my eggs. Usually, a woman has to take hormones for weeks or even months before having her eggs harvested, so hormones weren't an option.

Maybe in years to come, this might be one of the greatest discoveries of the century; however, something was telling me that I wasn't ready to have my reproductive organ stuffed into my limb. What if someone bumped into my arm? What would I say?

"Hey! Please be more careful. *That's* my ovary!"

I thanked "Dr. Frankenstein" for his time and walked out to the waiting room to my mom and Jennifer.

"How'd it go? What's the matter?" they both asked, perplexed.

"Come on, let's go," I whispered.

I threw my mother's pocketbook onto her arm and pushed them both out the door. I looked behind my shoulder in a panic as if, at any moment, a bolt of lightning would strike and "Frankenstein" would come walking out from the back room. We left as quickly as we came.

I decided to try another fertility doctor and, believe it or not, it was an even *worse* idea. My sister Theresa and I went together. Dr. Lee had me spinning in circles from the minute we arrived. She could have cared less that I had cancer; she just wanted me to get pregnant no matter how high the stakes.

After discussing several options, she told me that, if I immediately started hormone therapy, she just might be able to extract anywhere from eight to 12 eggs. Then she asked if I was married.

"No, I'm not married, but I have a boyfriend."

She continued by asking questions about him.

"To increase the chances of your eggs surviving and the success of becoming pregnant in the future, you may want to think about fertilizing your eggs before freezing them. Do you think your boyfriend would be willing to give us a specimen so we can fertilize your eggs?"

"I'll speak to him about it."

She told me that they would do the fertilization separately, and freeze the embryos until I was ready for artificial insemination. I'd also have to pay storage fees for the embryos. Wow, paying rent for my kids before they're even born … *amazing!*

After the consultation, the assistant led me from Dr. Lee's office into the examining room. I put on a paper gown, lay on the table, and placed each foot into a stirrup.

Dr. Lee walked in and cut to the chase without making any small talk. She inserted a long instrument inside me for the sonogram. While moving it around, she hesitated for a moment.

"I see a growth on one of your ovaries."

Well, I had breast cancer so, of course, I should have ovarian cancer, too.

"Oh, my God." I thought. "The cancer has spread to my ovaries!"

"You do?" I said anxiously, as I pressed both my feet against the stirrups.

She calmly continued by saying that it could be a harmless cyst related to my period.

I thought, "Harmless cyst? I've heard *that* one before."

Dr. Lee told me to wait until I got my period, which was due next week, and then come back in on that day. Most likely the cyst would be gone by then, so she'd have a better idea of what it might be.

I got dressed, thanked the good doctor, and quickly left with my sister.

As we walked through the halls and out the door, Theresa kept asking me what was wrong. She looked extremely worried and concerned. After I told her, we both became very quiet.

Unconvincingly, she said, "I'm sure it's nothing."

The following day, Peter and I went out to dinner with Jennifer and her husband. We were all drinking and having a great time, and joking about the fertility situation. The table then quieted down and everyone became serious.

Peter turned to me and said, "You can use my sperm to fertilize your eggs if you want."

I gave him a kiss, and then we all lifted up our glasses in a toast to our unborn babies. It didn't take long before the table filled up again with laugher and jokes. *Cheers!*

The following week, on Friday morning, I was supposed to go to the park for a picnic with friends. I got my period that morning, so I called the fertility clinic as they had instructed. They said to come in immediately so they could retest me for that growth.

I threw on my clothes and ran out the door without saying a word to anyone. I didn't want anybody to worry. I figured they would tell me that everything was okay and I would be home before they even missed me.

I arrived at Dr. Lee's office and again lay on the examining room table. She moved the instrument around in a circle, and then looked up from the draped paper blanket, which lay across my shaking knees.

The suspicious growth hadn't gone away. She told me there was a strong possibility that it could be ovarian cancer. In an instant, I went from pregnancy to *ovarian cancer*.

After telling me this, she started hounding me to start hormone therapy immediately so my eggs could be retrieved.

"I just want to go home," I repeated over and over.

"Well, if it *is* ovarian cancer, you wouldn't want to postpone retrieving your eggs, would you?"

84

After stalling for some time, she finally left the room and allowed me to get dressed. I slowly climbed down from the table, like a defeated soldier. The last bullet just pierced my heart. My legs were weak and my body was trembling. I put on my clothes and walked straight out of the office. I could see the doctors and nurses staring at me as I walked out.

It's over. The cancer's now in my ovaries.

I walked towards my car in a panic. I called my mom from my cell phone as tears streamed down my cheeks. I choked on my words as I told her where I was and what the doctor had said.

"Just come home. Don't worry. We'll take care of it, okay? Just come home right now, Mary."

Almost hyperventilating, and practically unable to get the words out, I called Lisa. I explained why I wouldn't be able to meet her for lunch. When I got home, the front door opened immediately. I collapsed into my mother's arms and cried.

She squeezed me tightly and repeated, "Don't worry, it'll be okay. We'll take care of it, okay?"

I slowly peeled myself out of her arms and walked up the stairs to my bedroom.

Not long after, Lisa and Peter showed up. My father began to call different doctors; however, it was late on a Friday afternoon and difficult to get in touch with anyone.

Theresa called and, when my mom picked up the phone, she walked into the other room to talk to her. I could hear my sister screaming through the phone. My mother kept telling her to calm down.

"Theresa," she said loudly, "stop it! Theresa, I said *stop* it! She'll be okay. Now *stop* it!"

I don't know what she was saying, but she was clearly upset.

Several hours passed and Peter had to leave to go to work. After I sat quietly with Lisa for a few minutes, she asked to take me for a ride. We wound up at a local beach—my favorite beach, where Peter took me when I first found out that I was sick. Not many words passed between us on the ride there.

We quietly got out of the car and began to walk towards the ocean. We stopped where the water met the sand and stood there motionless. As our hair blew in the air, we looked into the sky towards the horizon. The sun was beginning to set.

People talk about their lives flashing before them, and that was precisely what was transpiring at that very moment. I looked across the sand and water, and up to the white clouds against the orange sky. My life—what it was and what it would never become—played repeatedly in my head.

The next day, my parents took me to my aunt's gynecologist for a second opinion. It would be an entire week before a specialist from Sloan would be able to see me, and I needed to know now. I was frantic.

Dr. Limmer dimmed the lights as he sat down on a stool at my feet, disappearing from view behind the blanket across my legs. He pulled the cart with the monitor on it towards him as he inserted the sonogram instrument inside me. After a minute or two, his face popped up from behind the blanket to tell me that what he saw did not resemble cancer *whatsoever.*

My eyes welled up. After finishing, he stood up and told me that, within a couple of weeks, it should be gone and not to worry about it. If I were ever going to throw a doctor to the ground, jump on top of him, and kiss him, it would have been Dr. Limmer—without a doubt!

I controlled myself and shook his hand as I thanked him repeatedly. I walked out of the office with a feeling of rebirth.

Maybe I do have a fighting chance!

CHAPTER 11

Wigwam

I was unsure about my choice for an oncologist and discouraged about the last one, but I still had an appointment with Dr. Andrea, whom Dr. Bogen had recommended. One thing was certain: I would lose my hair from the chemotherapy.

Before I started any treatments, Lisa planned a "wig dinner" in my honor—a great attempt to make light of something that would end up weighing so heavily on me. It was a huge success.

Initially, a few of us met at my house; the others planned to meet us at a local Mexican restaurant. Everyone was standing around in my kitchen, laughing and chatting about what the evening had in store for us.

I opened a present from my friend Kristina: a "Dorothy" wig from *The Wizard of Oz*. I put it on and everyone giggled. Over the years, I made home movies with family and friends and collected a box full of wigs. I placed the large cardboard box in the middle of the kitchen for everyone.

Kate's husband Steve was the first to dig in and pull out a wig. Even though he mistakenly put it on upside down, I knew exactly which one it was—my Elvis wig, of course! Everyone burst out laughing.

"Oh, man! Okay, okay, I'll *wear* it!" he said, as he laughed uncontrollably.

Then Kate pulled a black, frizzy, curly wig over her platinum blonde hair. We all roared with laughter as her blonde hair fell out from under the black wig.

My brother-in-law Stephen tucked a snug, short, black, ratty wig on top of his head and looked just like a troll doll. He ran to bathroom to admire

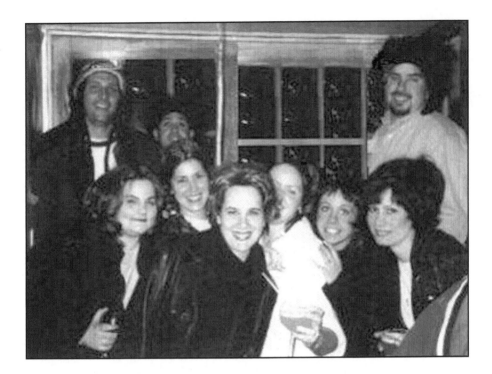

himself as everyone laughed and pointed at his head. There was no holding back. Everyone was poking fun and laughing at each other.

Then Margaret tucked and tucked and tucked her long, thick hair high into a short, black wig. Her head looked so pointy that everyone began calling her Conehead!

Ann Marie and her husband Frank showed up shortly thereafter. Frank walked in first, wearing a short, curly, platinum blonde wig like Marilyn Monroe. Then, Ann Marie followed in her long, red-haired wig. Peter put on a short, auburn wig—nicely styled, if I say so myself. Lisa was wearing a short, black wig, which actually didn't look half bad.

Elvis was laughing at Conehead, Conehead was laughing at The Troll, and The Troll was poking fun at Marilyn. It was hysterical!

When everyone had arrived at my house, it was time to leave. Fifteen of us were going out to dinner.

My friend Christine and her husband Billy were the first couple to arrive at the restaurant. Billy was wearing a Jamaican hat with dreadlocks hanging down, and Christine was wearing a long, black, straight wig over her long, curly, blonde hair. While waiting for everyone else, Billy happened to catch the attention of an African American gentleman. As the man walked passed, he stopped and turned towards Billy.

"Cool locks, dude!" the man said.

They both looked at one another and laughed.

Everyone gathered at the back entrance of the restaurant because no one had enough courage to walk through the front door. Our faces were red from embarrassment, and we hung our heads in shame.

Single file, we slowly walked through the door.

The place was jam packed. As large as the restaurant was, it was difficult to move because there were people standing around, waiting to be seated. We congregated around the door, either sitting or standing up against one another.

Naturally, our table wasn't ready; it would never be that easy. In sync, we swung around our wig heads and walked back out to the atrium to wait. We stood shoulder to shoulder, looking around impatiently and waiting for them to call us.

Every so often, we'd tug at our wigs, scratch our heads, or stuff a few hairs back into our wigs. All the while, we were trying to look comfortable and fit in with the dinner crowd so we wouldn't attract too much attention. It may have been embarrassing for my friends and family, but they were doing it for me. They were trying to make me laugh and keep my spirits up.

It was tough making conversation and acting cool, looking the way we did. I glanced over at Steve, with that large Elvis wig sitting on his head. It was also tough looking at Stephen The Troll, watching him nonchalantly looking around, trying to look like he was cool, calm, and relaxed.

One brave soul wandered off to the back of the restaurant and spotted the bar. It wasn't long before everyone began to light up again. We pushed and shoved our way through the crowd towards the booze. This short trip to the back of the restaurant was not as easy as it sounds.

We passed a woman in the crowd, who made a comment about Conehead Margaret. I saw the woman pointing at my sister.

She turned to another woman beside her and whispered, "My, that woman has an oddly shaped skull."

My sister and I looked at each other and laughed.

"It's a wig … a *wig*!" we shouted, but the woman must have known.

Kate tried to tuck her hair back under her wig as she made her way through the crowd. She kept turning around to me, laughing and grabbing onto my shoulder because I don't think she knew what to do with herself. Everyone was looking at us … I'd look at us, too!

We were making our way over to the bar when a woman turned to Kate, grabbed her arm, and commented on Steve's hair.

"Please tell me that's not his *real* hair! No one should have to go through life with hair like *that*!"

The woman had to have known that it was an Elvis wig. How could you not? It even had the thick sideburns, which, at this point, seemed to be curling up, giving it a "winged" effect on both sides of his head.

Kate didn't know what to say, so she nodded and smiled, and turned to me hysterically laughing as we continued the walk of shame.

Finally, we were seated, and it couldn't have been soon enough. We immediately ordered pitchers of sangria. I sat at the head of the table. It was great seeing my family and friends, each with a horrible wig resting on top of his/her head. It didn't take us very long to settle in, eat, drink, and be merry! We quickly became extremely comfortable with our new locks.

Our waitress brought over maracas and sombreros to add to the Mexican festivities. I threw one of the sombreros on top of my Dorothy wig.

"*Ole!*"

During dinner, I had to go to the bathroom. Peter escorted me to ensure that I made it there safely since I was a bit intoxicated.

I staggered to the door and, all of a sudden, I don't know what came over me. I grabbed his arm and, both laughing, pulled him into the ladies bathroom. Suddenly, I turned to the side and saw someone else opening the door and entering.

I looked up at Peter and then over to the bathroom stall behind us. The person was just about in the room, so I quickly threw him into the stall. Without hesitation, I dove in behind him and closed the latch.

I threw my hand over his mouth because he wasn't able to stop laughing out loud. We were both wearing our wigs and I still wore the sombrero. The brim was so big that it almost reached from one side of the tiny stall to the other. It was the toilet bowl, Peter, and me.

We heard a few more girls walk in, discussing how the only stall in the bathroom—other than the one we were in—*was stopped up and not working.*

This was a defining moment.

A crowd of girls began to line up outside, commented about the wait, and told me to hurry.

A short time later, to our surprise and in the midst of all the confusion, we heard someone step into the "stopped-up" stall next to ours. Her shoes squeaked on the wet floor as she walked in, turned around, and made herself at home. The door swung shut and the lock snapped closed.

I could hear a pocketbook being thrown up on the hook and bouncing off the side of the door. From what I had originally seen, there was no toilet paper in the dispenser because it was probably all in the bowl! This was beginning to get very interesting.

I looked down and saw her legs swaying. Her feet were tipping forward, backward, and then a little from side to side as if to balance. She was probably assuming "the stance," hovering over the toilet bowl, just about to pee.

Without warning, we heard an enormous downpour. The loud gush hit the stuffed-up toilet paper lodged in the bowl. It sounded like Niagara Falls smashing against a mountain of rocks.

I guess we kept the ladies waiting a little *too* long.

Men always wonder what goes on inside a woman's bathroom. Well, boys, it takes just a few short moments to pee, wash up, reapply make-up, and gossip. God forbid there's a broken toilet to put a halt in our routine. We'll just make do with what we have. Whether we need to stitch a tear in our dress with a portable sewing kit, hairspray our running pantyhose, or utilize a clogged toilet bowl.

Peter and I heard a loud voice coming from the "stopped-up" stall.

"Christine, I'll be right out!"

We looked at each other with puzzled faces. Instantaneously, we pointed towards the stall and mouthed two words at the same time.

"It's *Margaret!*"

My particularly clean sister, who doesn't go a day without cleaning her house, was the one peeing in that dirty stall!

I poked my head out the door and saw a very long line of girls, which continued out into the hall. Immediately, I pulled my head back in and slammed the door shut. Peter burst out laughing and couldn't control himself, so I kept flushing the toilet to try and drown him out. I burst out laughing myself, and smacked my hand over his mouth as he threw his hand over mine.

"Shhhhh," we softly said to one another.

We tried to hold back laughter, but the more my sister peed, the louder we got. After she was done, there was complete silence. Then, she must have realized that there was *no toilet paper*. I saw her feet shuffle forward and heard her digging around her pocketbook, looking for a tissue. Every woman probably has a crumpled-up, sneezed-on, lipstick-doused tissue *somewhere* in her pocketbook.

We finally heard the stall door swing open. After a while, many angry and frustrated girls left and the coast did finally clear. We waited until the last person left, and then Peter ran out and into the men's bathroom.

In the meantime, I walked back to my friends and family, who were still seated at the wig table. I slurred a confession about what had just happened, and everyone seemed to have a take on the story. They thought some hanky panky was going on in the old ladies' room bathroom stall, which couldn't have been further from the truth!

Everyone waited in anticipation for Peter to return to the table. When he did, we took a bow and were applauded and commended for our venture. It's funny how the silliest things in life can make our family and friends proud.

When it was finally time to go shopping for a real wig, Lisa offered to take me to a salon that received donated wigs from different charitable organizations. In an attempt to ease my nerves, she bought me a small bottle of liquor. Lisa thought that I needed a good buzz to try on fake hair and she was right. I looked like a dirty lush, tipping my head back and gripping the small liquor bottle wrapped in a tiny brown bag, but it didn't faze me. I sucked the bottle dry.

We walked into the salon in search of my new hair. I was courageous enough to try on several wigs, but the wigs this salesperson pulled out were disgraceful. To this day, I still think they were dirty brown mops—without the sticks. It didn't take very long for my eyes to well up with tears.

"Well, they were at the bottom of my closet," the salesperson said. "They'll look pretty after I wash and cut them."

"I don't look very pretty at all," I thought. "I'm sure it'll take more than just a wash and cut to do it."

The minute Lisa realized that I was getting upset, she yanked me out of the chair and literally threw me out the door, thanking the woman for her time and pushing me from behind. I know she felt bad and even offered to take me to a few other places, but all I really wanted to do was go home.

A few weeks later, Lisa took me to another place that was great. Kathleen, one of the owners, handled my situation very professionally. She took us into a back room and sat me in a beautician's chair. She placed wig after wig on me until I found one that was just right. She explained that, since I hadn't lost my hair yet, the wig would look even better once I did because the wig would actually hug my head.

After resembling Cousin It from *The Addams Family*, a shaggy rock star, a pageboy, and a variety of other characters, I finally picked out my wig. In fact, I liked it better than my real hair! Without hesitating, I bought it.

Maybe this wig thing won't be so bad after all?

CHAPTER 12

The Red Devil

y parents and I arrived early in the morning at the Breast Center to meet with an oncologist. Sloan–Kettering has an entire floor dedicated to the treatment of breast cancer.

Dr. Andrea walked into the examining room and shook my hand. After the customary polite introductions, she casually sat down on the tall biohazard container, positioned directly in front of the examining table where I sat. Both my mom and my dad were sitting off to the side. She began reading from a stack of papers—my personal file, I presumed.

Dr. Andrea was soft spoken, gentle, and kind; however, my guess is that the other doctors probably forewarned her: *"Caution: Contents under pressure … may explode at any time."*

She looked at me with her sweet face.

"Many times, cancer can be more aggressive in younger patients."

"Lovely. Already off to a good start," I thought.

I grabbed onto the sides of the table beneath me as my dangling legs began to tighten up. Tiny black dots formed in front of my eyes, and I felt faint as the flickering dots moved all around.

She said that I had 22 positive lymph nodes and described the type of treatments I would get. She suggested that I take part in a clinical trial and, if I consented to participate in the study, I would be randomly selected for one of three "arms" in the trial. Herceptin would be administered either along with the traditional chemotherapy regimen (for a few months during and/or after) or for an entire year preceding it. After explaining the risks of the clinical trial, she asked if I wanted to participate.

Everyone looked over at me.

The pressure was on.

As I sat there, pale with fear, I was in no condition to make that kind of decision. At that moment, if asked, I wouldn't be able to choose between a scoop of chocolate or vanilla ice cream.

I looked at her and thought, "You're kidding, right? Make a *decision*? Well, you're the doctor. Can't you make the decision *for* me?"

I knew that she wouldn't and neither would my parents. It was painfully obvious that it was entirely up to me, so I casually shrugged my shoulders.

"Okay, then. I'll just do it," I answered, as if I had just agreed to participate in a game of tennis.

I didn't give much thought to it because I didn't think it needed much thought. This was something that would help me and could even help others. The chemotherapy alone could pose many risks—never mind this clinical trial. I'd have to take my chances.

Dr. Andrea needed to place my name into a random drawing so that the database would decide whether I would receive the medication during my chemo, for six months after my chemo, or for an entire year following my chemo. Let the chips fall where they may.

She left the room for a while and, upon returning, said that I was accepted into the trial to receive weekly infusions for one year after chemotherapy. Furthermore, my treatments would begin on May 14th.

Dr. Andrea introduced me to Katherine, her head nurse. Katherine had me laughing from day one. She was Dr. Andrea's sarcastic sidekick, with that smirky smile of hers. She always looked like the cat that ate the mouse. Dr. Andrea also introduced me to Sandy, who was like the kindhearted girl next door. The three of them were just what I needed to get me through the upcoming months.

After the consultation, Dr. Andrea sent my parents and me into another room to speak with Katherine. She explained what was going to happen to me over the next year and a half.

The staff at Sloan would give me aggressive chemotherapy treatments for six months, followed by one month of radiation and a year of the clinical trial.

Katherine explained how the chemo would almost certainly make me nauseous. I would get medication before each treatment to try to prevent it, and even more meds to take home with me.

She said that my hair would definitely fall out and, when it did, it would go fast. It would most likely begin falling out about two weeks after the first treatment.

My blood count would be at its lowest about 10 to 14 days after treatments, so I'd have to be careful with germs, particularly around this time. On occasion, they could possibly admit me into the hospital for antibiotics if I got any infections.

Mouth sores, diarrhea, constipation, aches, pains, etc. It may be bad, but Katherine stressed that there is medicine to help with almost everything, so she encouraged me to tell her if anything was bothering me during the treatment.

"You don't need to suffer, Mary."

I quickly grew to love my sweet oncologist, her wise-ass nurse, and the cute girl next door. I went home to soak up all of the information given to me that day. It would be a bitter battle, but I was determined to prevail.

May 13th came quickly—the night before my first chemo treatment. I was in my bedroom when I heard a knock at the door. It was my dad. I was sitting on the floor, shuffling through my CDs, when he walked in. Before speaking, he hesitated and looked down at me.

"Listen," he said. "What you're about to go through is going to take a lot of courage. Now, I know you've got what it takes to do it, but you're going to have to try to stay strong, okay?"

I lifted my head to look at him and nodded.

"Okay, Dad. I will. I promise."

That was a poignant moment for me. I always looked up to and respected my father. If I made a promise to him, I had to stand by my word, and here he was, telling me that I needed to fight for my life. I would try as I promised, but I really didn't know if I actually could *do* it. I think he knew it, but that was what this talk was all about: a promise to fight like hell.

We looked each other in the eyes to say what we needed to say, but we truthfully didn't know if I would win or lose. Like a child, promising her daddy that she would be a good girl, would not talk to strangers, or would not cross the street without looking first, I promised my father that I would fight for my life.

I woke up early the next morning trembling. I had no idea what to expect. In the past, I had always been very sensitive to medication, and I was terrified that something like "chemotherapy" might do more than just kill cells … it might kill *me*.

After my parents and I arrived at Sloan, we waited for some time before we saw Dr. Andrea. She examined me quickly and then sent us back to the waiting room.

Before long, I heard, "Stolfa? Mary Stolfa?"

I met two technicians—Madge and Jack—who would take my blood count reading for the next year and a half by sticking my finger before each chemo treatment. Not long after that, someone else called me in for my first treatment.

I walked into one of the 20 or so small treatment rooms, each furnished with a counter, a small table, shelves, a recliner, and a TV, and sat quietly in the chair. I wanted to show my parents that I was ready to take it all in stride. I stretched out my arm and pushed up my sleeve.

"I *can* do this," I thought, as I firmly clenched my teeth.

Then, "Take It All in Stride" Mary looked down and saw her arm uncontrollably shaking.

I looked back up and focused straight ahead at the wall, waiting for them to begin my treatment. I was petrified. What will it be like? How will it make me feel?

Then, one of the technicians walked into the treatment room—one of the many nice techs who would administer the chemo throughout the course of my treatments. She was so sweet, with blonde hair, blue eyes, and an enchanting smile. All of the technicians seemed to possess the same angelic appearance.

"Hi, Mary," she said. "My name's Linda."

After a few small pleasantries, she set up my IV line and explained what was about to happen. She handed me six pills to take, mostly for nausea. After watching her pull needles, tubes, and IV lines out of the cabinets, and then walking in and out of the room several times, I finally got the nerve to ask her a couple of questions as I trembled in my seat.

As frightened as I was, I politely asked, "Linda, when might I get the medicine that Dr. Andrea was talking about a little earlier? You know … the medicine that will help me calm down a little?"

"Of course, Mary. I'll get that for you right now. Don't worry."

She firmly held my quivering arm as she inserted the IV line. The saline solution felt cold running through my veins—almost like ice water. After that ran for several minutes, she injected something else into the line. Within seconds, my body stopped shaking so much.

Another nurse walked in to double check my name and the medication, which would become the standard routine before every treatment to make sure that I wasn't getting someone else's medication by accident. One less thing for me to worry about, I guess.

Linda got three 6-inch red needles, filled with Adriamycin—the "Red Devil"—and sat down on a stool right next to me. This medication is the driving force behind most of the sickness, nausea, vomiting, and every other repulsive side effect of the chemo. I quickly learned how the "Red Devil" got its nickname.

I watched as Linda slowly injected these three needles directly into the IV line. It took minutes for the first medication to be administered. I sat there for another hour while Cytoxin, the rest of the treatment, was infused.

After my treatment was finally over, my parents each took one of my arms and together we all walked out to the car. I lay down on the back seat because I was starting to feel a little queasy. On the way home, I heard my parents talking about all of the cancer-fighting, antioxidant, healthy food they would make me for dinner.

As my stomach began turning, my parents continued to chat about the huge steak they were going to make for me when we got home ... and broccoli, lots and lots of broccoli. I popped up my head and stuck it between their two seats.

"You've *got* to be kidding," I said, and then slipped into unconsciousness.

Regardless of all the pills I was taking over the next few days, I was sick anyway. The pills were supposed to alleviate the vomiting somewhat, but they didn't seem to be helping very much at all. In fact, they gave me *other* side effects, so I eventually stopped taking them altogether.

In between the nausea waves during the first week, I had cravings for pizza. I made the mistake of telling my dad that I was in the mood for a "middle" slice of Sicilian pizza. My poor dad went to three pizzerias before finding one that had what I wanted. The first two didn't have any of those slices left. He finally came home with two middle slices of Sicilian pizza for his little girl.

The nausea bout lasted about a week and a half after my treatment. Then I started to feel a little better and, that weekend, wound up at a comedy club in New York City with Peter and friends. Before we left, I wasn't feeling very well, but I didn't want to worry anyone. By the time we got home from the club, I was extremely dizzy and very sick. I went straight to bed, knowing that something was seriously wrong. I woke up the next morning and noticed that the gum near my wisdom tooth had swelled. I was in excruciating pain and unable to close my mouth.

It was Sunday, so my mom had to call Sloan's emergency number to speak with the doctor on call. He told me to take my temperature because a temperature usually indicates an infection. I had a mild fever, so he instructed me to go to a local emergency room since Sloan was about an hour away. My mom, dad, and I left immediately.

Even though the waiting room was crowded, they called me in relatively quickly to see the doctor. After running numerous blood tests, the nurse walked over and told me that it shouldn't be a problem to go home. She was a friend of the family and didn't want to alarm us. The results from the tests weren't in yet, but she didn't foresee any problems.

Just as I was about to hop off the table and leave, the phone in the ER rang. In the midst of examining other patients, the doctor answered it and looked over at me as he spoke. After a few minutes, he hung up and headed towards us.

My heart started to pound out of my chest and I took a deep breath; my arms and legs tightened as he walked over. I was terrified of what he was going to tell me.

"What *is* it? Is he going to tell me that I'm dying?" I wondered.

"Your blood count is .1," the doctor said. "That's very low. I just spoke with the doctor on call in the emergency room at Sloan and he requested that you come right in."

We immediately left for New York City.

I was petrified as we walked into the emergency room entrance. They called me in right away, told me to lie on the bed behind one of the 10 or so curtains, and hooked me up to an IV line. The nurse drew tube after tube of blood as my parents stood and watched.

Numerous doctors and nurses walked in and out, asking me all sorts of questions while pushing, poking, pressing, and scoping every part of my body. At one point, a group of doctors walked in with my chart and discussed my diagnosis, treatment, and status—talking about me as if I weren't even there.

I lay back as they pushed and tapped on my stomach. They pressed every inch of my body, asking if it hurt.

They continued their conversation in "doctor talk" with their fancy schmancy words, felt my glands, and shined lights into my eyes and down my throat—not acknowledging the fact that I was more than just *cancer*.

All of a sudden, I burst out crying, and the doctors were quickly escorted out by the attending doctor. Then, the attending doctor came through the curtain, rushed over to my mom and dad, and explained that they were just students.

He took my hand and apologized that they had upset me, but I had already come to my own conclusion: We were playing *The Price Is Right*. Behind Curtain #1 was a brand new car, behind Curtain #2 was a brand new washer and dryer, and behind Curtain #3 was a dying patient. I was behind Curtain #3.

I was scared, confused, and didn't understand what was happening. I thought they were lying to me so I wouldn't be scared that the cancer had already spread. I thought that was the reason why my blood count was so low.

My dad left for a while, and my mom sat on the chair next to my bed.

I heard one of the nurses say, "She's over there."

I looked up and saw a smiling Peter peek through the curtains. He walked in and gave me a big kiss. Both he and my dad always had the "everything's going to be fine, what are you so worried about?" look; on the other hand, my mom and I always had the "I am so freakin' worried that I don't know what to do with myself" look.

Not long after, my dad came back with an angel pin for me. He put it on my hospital gown, and pressed the button that made the little lights around it flicker.

"That's for my little angel," he said and smiled.

One of the doctors walked in to tell me not to worry. He was very nice. He said that I had an infection in my mouth, so I'd have to be admitted. By staying a few days, they could administer antibiotics intravenously to cure the infection. He told me not to worry and that they were going to take very good care of me.

That night, my mom stayed with me. I begged her to keep the snoring engine down this time. Once again, she made her makeshift bed in the chair, and we both dozed off with the TV on.

I woke up in the middle of the night, looked over at my mom's chair, and it was empty. I glanced towards the bathroom, but the door was open and the light was off. I thought she may have gone to the bathroom down the hall or maybe for a walk. After a while, I began to worry.

I grabbed my IV pole and went searching for her. I checked the lounge on my floor and all the bathrooms, but I couldn't find her anywhere. I even asked the nurses at the front desk if they had seen her roaming around. They hadn't, but they told me that there was another lobby downstairs on the main floor.

I took the elevator down to the lower level. The doors opened into a dark, quiet hallway. I slowly wheeled my IV pole towards the dimly lit, huge, empty lounge area. I was barely able to make out the many rows of empty seats.

When I got to the lounge entrance, I stopped to look around. I walked inside and looked down each aisle. The only thing I could hear was the echo from the wheels of my IV pole as I pulled it along.

Then I spotted her. As I slowly walked over, I was just about able to make out the top of her head. She was slumped in the chair, half-asleep, trying to read her angel book.

"What are you doing here, Mom?"

"Just reading," she said. "I didn't want to keep you awake with my snoring."

"*What?* Please go to bed!"

I took her hand and we both walked back to my room together.

The next day, doctors came in and out of my room. Every time I saw a group walk in (and they were *always* in groups), I'd get a pit in my stomach. I kept thinking that they were coming to give me some sort of bad news. The furthest thing from my mind was that they were coming in to examine me. I mean, after all, I *was* in a hospital.

Later that day, I went to an oral surgeon in the hospital for the swelling in my mouth, but it was completely unnecessary because I had already come up with a diagnosis myself: *mouth cancer*, of course.

After taking a few x-rays, Dr. Posa told me that my wisdom tooth was slowly breaking through my gum, allowing bacteria to get in, which was causing the infection, so he would remove the tooth the next morning.

"Tooth? Infection? Okay, if you say so," I thought, "but don't say I didn't warn you when it turns out to be *cancer*."

Dr. Posa took off his rubber gloves and started to wash his hands. As he reached for the paper towels, he leaned towards me.

"Do you wanna hear a secret?"

"Sure," I said. "About what?"

"It's about your family."

"Uh, oh. What'd they do now?"

"No, no," Dr. Posa said. "It's not like that. It's good! The entire hospital is talking about them. All of the nurses and doctors keep saying how nice your entire family is. Everyone adores all of you."

"Wow! I am absolutely flattered. Well, I also have to say that my entire family thinks very highly of all of you. Everyone has been so kind to us. Thank you so much for everything."

Throughout the night and the following day in the hospital, I continued to receive antibiotics and injections to increase my white blood cell count. About two days after my admittance, my hair began to fall out, and I found strands all over my bed and pillow. As the day went on, I seemed to be shedding more and more. It began to come out in fistfuls, and I wasn't able to run my fingers through it without removing a handful of hair.

My mom decided to call the hospital "beautician" to come and give me a haircut. When the woman arrived, she suggested shaving it all off.

"We'll just take the rest of it off since there really isn't much left to shape."

I was heartbroken. I knew the time would come, but I wasn't as prepared as I thought I would be.

All along, I kept thinking, "It's only hair. It'll grow back. It's no big deal."

Even though my hair had thinned out with large bald patches, and although there were just leftover straggles dangling from my head, the thought was still tremendously painful. It wasn't easy to let it go. When the beautician told me that it was time to shave it off, I sunk into my bed and tears quickly welled up in my eyes.

I looked down at the sheets and said, "Okay, then … whatever you think."

I slowly got up from bed as the beautician and my mom struggled to grab a chair in the corner for me. The beautician plugged her electric shaver into the outlet and took a pair of scissors from her bag. I sat on the chair and looked straight ahead.

This was going to be a "triumph" for me—not a "trial." I had come so far, and I wasn't going to let the hair on my head get me down. Like Samson, with every bit of courage and strength I had, I was going to defeat this enemy that wanted my life as well as my will and spirit to live. I kept telling myself that I was bigger, stronger, and more powerful than what anyone put before me.

My roommate and new friend Shelly, who was receiving massive doses of chemo for ovarian cancer, sat on her bed and read a book. I looked past her and stared at the back wall. My eyes glazed over, but I could still see her silhouette off to the right.

As the beautician continued to set up, I tried incredibly hard to hold back my tears but, all of a sudden, they began to gush down my face. I kept trying to "swallow" the hurt, gulp after gulp, but I just couldn't do it. I repeated to myself how my hair didn't matter, and all that *did* matter was that I got better, but the emotional pain was unbearable.

Through the ocean of tears, I saw Shelly look at me, close her book, get up, and sadly leave the room. My mom took the hat, which my sister Margaret had left for me, and placed it on the bed next to her. She cried as she sat there and watched.

The beautician grabbed a fistful of hair. With her scissors and one big *swoosh*, she chopped it off. She continued around my head, snipping away at any leftover stragglers. I froze in my seat and wouldn't move my head. From the corner of my eyes, I barely saw the beautician reach for the electric razor—the "buzzer."

Click.

I quietly sobbed as she pressed the buzzer against my head, its loud screech piercing my heart. I'll never forget what it felt like to have that buzzer press against my head. With each stroke, it got louder and my head would push forward; with each stroke, I would weep even more.

After the beautician finished, both she and my mom quickly threw a hat on top of my head. After they swept the floor, the beautician left. I quietly cried to my mother as she hugged me tightly. She told me over and over how beautiful I still looked, but I certainly didn't *feel* beautiful.

I got back in bed and fell asleep for a while. I was just beginning to wake up when I heard my mom outside the door.

"Did you see her yet?"

I opened my eyes and saw my dad walking towards me. I waited impatiently for his response.

"You look like a little kid!" he said, with a great big smile as he kissed me.

My hospital floor was like no other. It had wallpaper, and TVs and VCRs were in every room. A beautifully decorated lounge occupied the middle of the floor, with its own TV, computer, couches, table, and chairs. In fact, if it weren't for the whole "sick cancer" thing, the floor might have made for a pleasant stay!

It would have also helped to have a better activities coordinator (like Julie McCoy from *The Love Boat*) than the floor nurse, who poked you with needles all day and all night.

A little while later, a waiter walked into my room. (Yes, a *waiter* ... to take my *order!*) He handed me an enormous menu, with choices such as hamburgers, pasta, omelets, and sundaes—anything you could ever want from soup to nuts.

I was in somewhat better spirits, so I ordered a bacon cheeseburger, sweet potato French fries, and ice cream. I ate like a queen! After finishing my dinner, I lay back in bed to digest all of that good hospital food. (It's strange to use "good" and "hospital food" in the same sentence.)

That night, family and friends came to visit. They surrounded my bed and chatted amongst themselves. I turned to the side and saw Peter, who was coming straight from work and still in uniform. Everyone backed away so he could get through. This was the first time he'd see me bald.

As he made his way towards me, the noisy room instantly became silent. He walked up to my bed and stood there for a moment, looking down at me. He leaned over and gently held the brim of my hat. He tipped it back so he could see my face completely. My lower lip started to quiver, and I could feel myself just about ready to cry. I was ashamed and brokenhearted.

He bent over and kissed me four times: one cheek, then the other, then my chin, and lastly my forehead. The room was still, eagerly anticipating what he was going to say. He stepped back and took off his gun belt. A tremendous smile filled his face as he shrugged his shoulders.

"*What?* You look just as beautiful as you always did!"

Everyone, especially me, smiled. You could actually hear a sigh of relief in the room.

Things settled down and everyone, except Peter, left. My parents went to get a bite to eat. I sat up, swung my legs around, and positioned myself on the edge of the bed, facing him with my back to the door. We talked as he nibbled on my fancy food leftovers.

It started to get very hot for him in the room, especially with all of the equipment he was wearing, so he stood up and unbuttoned his shirt to get to his bulletproof vest. While watching the door behind me to make sure that no one was coming, he quickly pulled his shirt out from his pants, flung it off, ripped open his vest, and quickly put his shirt back on. With his bare chest bursting out, he unclipped his belt and unbuttoned his pants, so he could tuck his shirt back down into them. As he began to unzip his fly, I quickly looked down at the floor. I could feel my face turning bright red.

As I asked him how his day was, I unintentionally glanced up at the exact moment his pants lay wide open. My face was directly in front of his crotch, just inches away. Just as his hand was stretching down his boxers to tuck in his shirt, one of the nurses burst through the door.

"I just wanted to give you your medicine for …"

Peter looked up and I swung my head around. She walked in and, without stopping, turned completely around and quickly dashed back out.

We could hear "I am so sorry!" echoing as she raced down the hall.

I turned my head back around and innocently looked up at Peter. We both shrugged our shoulders, not understanding what had just happened. Then, all of a sudden, we realized what she was probably thinking.

"No, *wait!*" Peter shouted, as he zipped up his pants and ran after her. "Come back! It's not what you think!"

He caught up to her and she came back to give me my injection, but the three of us stood silently and blushed until she left the room.

The following morning, I saw Dr. Posa again because it was time for him to extract my tooth … and I thought the *mastectomy* was bad! After I sat down in the chair, and had a dribble bib hooked around my neck, Dr. Posa walked into the room. He had a confused look on his face.

"Hi?"

"Yeah, my hair's all gone."

"Wow! I *love* it! You look like Sinéad O'Connor!"

He was such a nice guy and kept cracking me up, but when it was time for that tooth to come out, he didn't hold any punches. My gums were overlapping the tooth, so it wasn't going to be an easy task getting it out. After injecting needle after needle of Novocain, this very nice oral surgeon reached over and thrust his entire fist into my mouth. He began to push, pull, dig and twist in all directions.

At one point, I looked up and saw veins popping out of his arms and face, as he continued ramming some wrench-like tool into my mouth. I thought my jaw would break in half with all the strength he forced down on me.

Sweat formed above his brows and his teeth gritted tightly together, almost as if he were competing in a game of tug-of-war, only it was my lonesome tooth against this six-foot-tall man and his wrench. Tears trickled out from the corners of my eyes, but I didn't want to complain.

"Are you okay, Mary?"

"I'm fine," I slurred, with my head jerking back and forth as he tugged at the tooth.

After a bitter battle, my tooth finally relinquished and came out. Dr. Posa sewed up the gaping hole and sent me back to my room.

My roommate Shelly brought movies to watch because she was there for a lengthy treatment. When I went back to the room, she popped a movie into the VCR to take my mind off the pain. Drool streamed out of my numb mouth as I fell asleep.

Not long after, Dr. Posa came to check on me. I heard him ask the nurses where I was because he only saw a little boy lying in the bed that they told him was mine.

"Little boy?" I thought. "Hey, you said that I was a beautiful, bald woman who looked like Sinéad O'Connor!"

As I slowly lifted up my head and nearly opened one eye, I saw him standing over my bed. He smiled, cracked a joke or two, and then threw a compliment out as he left.

I stayed in the hospital for a few more days until my blood count finally went back up. At home, I was sitting at the kitchen table, having something to eat, and the front door swung open.

My sister Bernie burst in. My parents had just picked her up from the group home where she lives during the week. She walked down the hallway and headed straight for the kitchen. It was the first time she was going to see me bald.

Upon entering the room, she stopped dead in her tracks. Bashfully, she made her way over to the counter but still kept her distance from me across the room. Unsure of what to do, she reluctantly walked towards me, but in midstream decided against it and backed up against the counter. With a huge smile that reached from ear to ear, she lifted both hands in front of her face and covered her eyes.

"Hi," she said apprehensively from behind 10 fingers.

"Hi, Bernie," I said, thinking that she was just uncomfortable with my new hairdo.

Shrugging her shoulders and tipping her head to the side, she politely spoke as she removed one hand from her face and extended it out to shake mine.

"What's *your* name?"

I suddenly realized that she had absolutely no idea who I was!

"Bernie, it's me. *Mary*! What's different about me?"

Her eyes suddenly lit up and opened wide in amazement. All of a sudden, she realized who I was.

"*Mary*! You got a haircut!"

"Do you like it?"

"Yeah, yeah, I do, Mary. *Cool, dude!*" she said happily, as she lifted her thumb up into the air to show her approval.

Later that night, I saw my three-year-old nephew Michael, also for the first time since I was bald. I was wearing my hat when he first arrived, and he started talking to me as if nothing were different. It's funny how a child doesn't judge someone on looks. I was the very same aunt to him.

I loved to make him laugh. Since I didn't get an initial reaction from my bald head, I decided to take my hat off and start making funny faces, and he laughed hysterically. From then on, it became our game. It was a big joke for him to be able to grab my hat, particularly when I was with a crowd of people so that I would get embarrassed. He'd tear it off my head and then run like

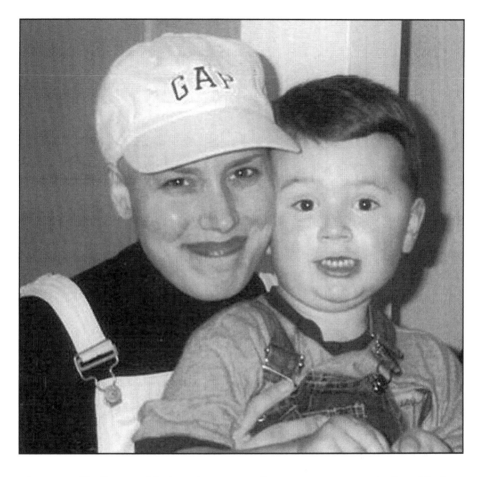

a bat out of hell! I would chase him around, trying to recover the hat. My face would turn red from shame and his red from laughter.

I was able to run after him on the good days but, as time progressed, the treatments were taking their toll and the sickness I would feel became stronger and lasted much longer.

Friends and family would visit and hop into bed with me or take me out when I was up to it. My friend Ann Marie would actually kneel at the side of my bed for hours and hold my hand.

Every organ in my body throbbed. At times, I was so brutally sick that I would just stay in the bathroom. I'd take a pillow in with me, keep the toilet seat up, curl up on the floor, and lie there for hours. Every so often, gathering what little strength I had, I'd lift up my head and vomit into the toilet bowl. I would flush, rinse out my mouth, and then fall back down onto the cold, ceramic floor. During the times when I didn't stay in the bathroom, I would run from my bedroom across the hall to and from it.

I got my cat Mary Ann 10 years ago, even though my mom didn't want a cat, and named her after my mom.

"Mary Ann, meet Mary Ann," I said with a grin, as I placed an adorable little fuzzy fur ball into my mother's arms.

How could she refuse?

Mary Ann stayed by my side and followed me back and forth when I got sick. I would jump out of bed and dash for the bathroom, and she would run alongside my feet. She stayed with me the entire time, sitting next to me when I lay my head on the side of the bathtub. I think she was watching to make sure I was okay.

Sometimes I would actually confide in Mary Ann, telling her how sick I felt and that I didn't know what to do to make it better. I cried, with my cheek pressed up against the ice cold side of the tub, and told her how I just wanted it all to stop.

She looked back at me and eventually stood up. She swayed her tail back and forth and then rubbed her soft, fluffy body against mine. If she had arms and could talk, I think she would have wrapped them around me and told me that everything was going to be fine.

When there was nothing left to come up—or at least I *thought* there was nothing left—I returned to my bed. Mary Ann snuggled up next to me, as I shivered under my covers. It lasted until the next bout when I raced to the bathroom once again.

I never had a cat before Mary Ann (we always had dogs), but I think Mary Ann came home with me that one night 10 years ago because she had a very important purpose to her life: I think she was sent to watch over me while I was getting sick. She stood beside me many times when I didn't want to upset anyone else.

Home wasn't the only place I was getting sick now; I was no longer able to make it back from chemo without vomiting. My mom and dad brought buckets in the car so we could pull over to the side of the road on short notice.

Every week, both of my parents would drive me all the way into the city for my chemo treatments. Sometimes it would be a 45-minute ride and sometimes three hours, depending upon traffic. Every week, they would prepare as if we were taking a cross-country trip!

They'd pack bags of quarters for the parking meters. My dad would load up the car with umbrellas, bags, paper towels, extra shirts, and other useless—I mean *useful*—stuff, and then fill it with gas.

My mom would put pillows, blankets, bottled water, crackers, gum, and other miscellaneous things aboard for our "big journey" into the city. You'd think we were driving all the way from good old New York to sunny California!

Every time I went for chemo, Peter—in his uniform—would also come to visit me during work. He, sometimes his partners, my parents, and friends and family would sit with me. It kept me occupied during my treatments.

One time, on the way home from a treatment, I was lying on the back seat as I usually did and felt a wave of nausea suddenly come over me. This was one time when I appreciated my parents' preparation.

I jumped up and asked my mom for a bucket. She quickly handed it to me as my dad swerved over to the curb. I threw open the door and dropped down to my knees. My mom held my head as I violently threw up. It actually felt as if my body were struggling to throw up a gigantic elephant. My face turned bright red, the veins in my neck blew up and pulsated, and my body trembled as I vomited off the side of the major highway.

It was never a normal kind of throwing up—at least not the "hangover" wine kind to which I was accustomed. I didn't have fun the night before, and the nausea didn't end in the morning.

It was the kind of throwing up and nausea that I think a person can only get from being pumped full of poison. It almost felt as if my body were trying to upheave my internal organs. I had many broken blood vessels in my eyes and all over my face from straining so hard.

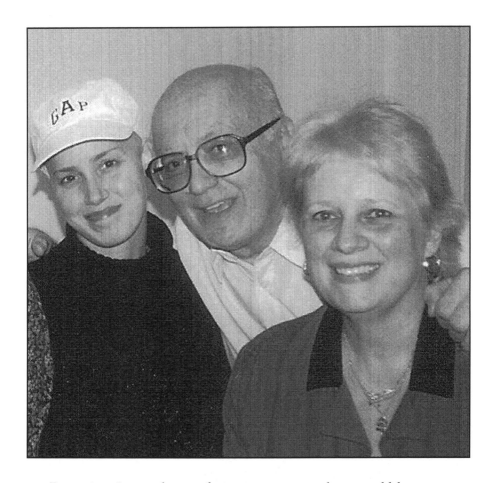

Every time I came home after my treatments, there would be a present waiting for me at my door. Peter would leave a card, a rose, and candy for me. No matter how horrible I was feeling, I was always able to muster a smile for his gifts as I walked in the door. Some days, I was too weak to pick them up and bring them in, so my mom or dad would do it; however, I would always open his card after I got in the door.

Peter told me many times while I was sick, "I always want to be able to see that wonder in your eyes."

He probably meant to say that he always wanted to be able to see that conniving smile, which made me look as if I were up to no good! Well, maybe he really *did* mean "wonder"—the wonder of what excitement the next day would bring, and the love for life that always shone through, which had probably been recently obscured by so much pain and suffering.

One day, when we were both lying on the couch watching TV, with Peter behind me, I began to cry.

"What's wrong, honey?"

As I started to sob, I said that I just couldn't do it anymore. I was too weak and too sick, and I didn't think I could go on.

He explained that it was either fight or give up, and he wasn't letting me give up any time soon. I had no choice. I needed to fight. I needed to go on. I needed to live. Then he wrapped his arms tightly around me and gently kissed the top of my bald head.

Many nights after I got my treatments, my body would shake uncontrollably for no apparent reason. One time, in the middle of the night, my mom crawled into bed with me, as she had done so many times before when the sickness got very bad. The lights were off and everything was quiet. I was awake but, after a while, my mom fell asleep.

All of a sudden, I heard a loud shriek, as if someone were trying to start a car. My air conditioner was directly above us, and its hum muffled the noise, but it sounded as if someone were repeatedly turning the ignition key and the motor wasn't starting up. After a few eruptions, I lifted my head and looked out the window.

"Who would possibly try to start their car again and again like that in the middle of the night?" I wondered.

I leaned over my mom and looked at the clock: 12:50 a.m.

As I reached back over her, I glanced down. I heard a loud snort come out of her mouth that made me cringe. Startled, I lay back down in disbelief. Of course—the "car" was my mom's snoring! I should have known.

It continued, quickly becoming heavier and louder. Before long, the "car" started, the engine was in full force, and it sounded as if an old, souped-up

Chevy Camaro were sitting right in the middle of my bedroom. However, it wasn't a monstrous engine; it was my mother.

I rolled over and tried to fall asleep for the next hour and a half. Every once in a while, I'd jab her with my arm in the hopes of stopping the snoring, but most of the time she'd stop for a split second, slither up her drool, and then fall back into the deep sleep that was producing that horrible noise. I was clearly *not* going to sleep any time soon, so I grabbed my pillow and slowly climbed over the big-engined car in an attempt to exit the garage.

As I lifted my leg into the air and carefully placed it down on the other side of her, she woke up. Not one move from all of my pokes, jabs, and pushes, but a subtle getaway attempt and she was all over me.

"What's the matter?" she said, as her eyes opened slightly.

"Nothing."

I jumped off the bed and hid my pillow from her view. There was a nightlight in the hallway, and I thought she might spot it.

"I'm just going to the bathroom, Mom."

I headed for the bathroom and waited inside for a few minutes before flushing and coming out. When I looked back in the room, there she was— revving the engine.

Now my pillow and I had to fend for ourselves, so I headed to my parents' room and slid into bed with my dad.

"Ah," I thought, "finally some peace and quiet."

There was silence for a brief moment as I snuggled under the blankets and closed my eyes. Then, with one very long breath, my father, too, burst into a thunderous snore. How in the world do the two of them ever get any *sleep*? It must be like the Indy 500 in their room every night!

I took my pillow and headed downstairs to the couch, where I slept the rest of the night. When dawn came, I snuck back upstairs and into my bed with my mom before she noticed that I was gone.

About a half hour later, she woke up and asked how I was feeling.

"A little better, thanks."

"Did you have a good night's sleep?" she asked.

"I had a good sleep. Thanks for staying with me last night, Mom."

There were many times, just like that night, when my mom stayed with me. There were also nights when I didn't want to worry her.

I loved to have angels around me and, over the years, I received many "angel" gifts, which I put in my bedroom. One night—a particularly bad night for me—I turned around in my bed, looked up at the ceiling, and saw a little cherub angel looking down at me. He was right above my face. I watched him slowly drift to the foot of my bed and then disappear.

Perhaps it was the chemo or a reflection in my eyes from outside. Whatever anyone else thinks, I truly believe that it was an angel.

I got a blood test before each one of my chemo treatments because my oncologist needed to check certain levels beforehand. On occasion, my counts would be so low that they had to postpone the treatment.

Each time I walked into the room to have either Madge or Jack take my blood, we always seemed to find something to amuse us. Despite how scared I was, we managed to crack a smile and tell a joke. My mother said that, as time went on, she'd hear roaring laughter coming from the room when I was in there with them.

The day finally came when I received my last Adriamycin and Cytoxin treatments. A few days later, my parents had to go upstate to Albany to take care of something for my father's business. That morning, my mom kept asking me if I would be all right to stay by myself until they got home. I told her that I was fine and not to worry. I didn't want my dad to have to go all by himself, so I told them repeatedly that I would be okay; however, I wasn't feeling well at all.

About an hour after they left, I got very sick, bent over with excruciating stomach pains. My body wouldn't stop shivering and I threw up more than usual. I felt as if I were dying. I could actually feel every organ inside of me writhing in agonizing pain. I curled into a ball on the couch and rocked myself back and forth.

"Please, my Lord. Please help me," I said, as I wrapped my arms tightly around my body. I clutched my rosary beads as I twisted and turned in every direction.

Not long afterwards, my mom called. I felt bad telling her about my condition, knowing very well that they weren't close and I would worry them, but I had to do it. I didn't know what else to do. I actually thought I was dying. A few minutes into the conversation, I blurted out how sick I really was. She immediately called my sister Margaret to have her stay with me until they got home.

Later, I found out how worried Margaret was when she saw how bad I looked that day, but she certainly didn't show it to me at the time. She was pregnant and kept showing me her belly to try to make me smile. In between flipping up her shirt, taking the measuring tape out and wrapping it around her waist, lying on the floor so I could examine the size of it, and swinging from side to side to show me her profile, she tried to get me to eat.

I just couldn't do it, though. My lips were purple and quivering, and I just lay there. My perspiring bald head was completely white and the circles around my eyes were almost black. I threw my rosary beads over my head to let them hang around my neck because I became too weak to hold them.

Before my parents made it home, Nicholas, Theresa, and my nephew Michael rushed over. Michael always had a way of cheering me up and making me feel better, but this time it wasn't working.

I pressed my face against the couch and everyone sat around me. They put a pillow underneath my cheek to prop me up. The rosary beads, which wrapped around my neck, draped over the side of the couch along with one of my arms. I just lay there, almost lifeless.

After a short while, Theresa nervously insisted that what I probably needed was some iron in my body. She dragged herself up from the couch and walked into the kitchen. I heard the freezer door fly open and slam against the cabinet beside it. After hearing things shuffle around, bags scrunch up, and something tumble across the kitchen floor, my sister appeared out of nowhere. She stood in front of me, holding a rather large frozen steak in both hands.

My eye—the one that wasn't squashed into the pillow—peeped out and spotted this humongous piece of meat suspended above my head.

"You need *meat!*" Theresa shouted. "Meat will make you feel better. There's iron in it!" she relentlessly said as she walked back into the kitchen.

Within minutes, I heard a loud bang. It must have been the massive steak hitting the frying pan because, seconds later, I saw smoke emerge from around the corner. Then I heard bang after bang, as my sister flipped the frozen piece of meat in the pan.

My parents arrived home shortly thereafter. I pulled myself up from the couch as my mom helped me over to the kitchen table. Everyone stood around as I forced a few pieces of steak into my mouth. Then, I went back to the couch and fell asleep.

I felt weak and shaky for weeks afterwards but never as bad as the day I thought I was going to succumb to the Red Devil.

CHAPTER 13

Hanging on by a Hair

When I lost my hair, it wasn't just on top of my head; eyebrow hairs, eyelash hairs, leg hairs, you name it—*every* hair fell out. I was most comfortable wearing baseball hats to cover my bald head; I saved my wig for dressier occasions when a hat wasn't appropriate.

People stared at me wherever I went. The bizarre part about it was that I really didn't care so much if they knew I had cancer, but I was way too vain to have them think that I was some kind of freak who decided to shave her hair and eyebrows. I couldn't have that.

One day, I went to the mall with my friend Ann Marie. We were casually walking along and minding our own business. She must have spotted someone staring at me because one minute she was beside me and then next minute she was out of sight.

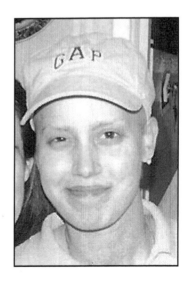

I quickly turned my head and saw her standing in the middle of the aisle, hands on hips, staring at a woman.

Embarrassed, I went over to her, looked down at the floor, and said, "Ann Marie, come on. Let's go. It's okay, let's just go."

Clearly ignoring me, she persisted in staring at this woman until the woman finally realized that she was being stared back *at*. The lady shamefully turned away.

I felt bad because I understood how people sometimes didn't realize what they were doing. Who knows? She might have had cancer at one time herself, or maybe she knew someone who did. Most people who passed me usually looked with empathy, but I didn't want anyone pitying me.

I know that Ann Marie was just defending me. She knew I was hurting and didn't want me to hurt anymore, but I just wanted to be another face in the crowd. I didn't want anyone to look at me differently, whether I was out in public or at parties with family and friends.

Throughout my chemo treatments, I received invitations to weddings and special occasions as I always had. As long as I was able to stand, I insisted on attending every one of them. I had a special need to go to these events, in spite of how sick I felt. In a way, I felt as though I were somehow getting back at the cancer. I think a part of me also didn't know if it would be the last event I would be able to attend. I had no idea what the future held.

The first wedding invitation I received prompted me to go shopping for a new dress. I needed something that would disguise the large tissue expander in my chest, which pushed upward, towards my collarbone, and looked extremely awkward—as if I had jammed a hockey puck underneath my skin.

Everyone offered to accompany me, but I decided to go to the department store myself, wearing my blue baseball hat and shirt to match. I was too anxious to bring anyone else and I needed to go alone.

I wandered around the Ladies Dress Wear section for some time. Every so often, I spotted customers or workers catching a glimpse of me. Finally, I picked a couple of dresses off the rack: two short cocktail dresses and a long, black one.

I walked into the dressing room and placed them on a hook. I took off my cap and threw it to the side. Then, I quickly took off my clothes and nervously kicked them into the corner on the floor.

I slid the first dress over my head. It was a short, black cocktail dress. On the left side of my chest, the tissue expander stuck straight out under my skin. On the right side of my chest, my real breast plunged south towards my foot.

121

The fluorescent lights were shining off my bald head. I looked in the mirror and then down at the floor.

It was repulsive.

I took the dress off and decided to try on the long, black one. This dress had a high neckline, almost like a priest's collar, and it draped down to the floor. Not particularly my style, but I figured it would cover as much of my body as possible, which had now become my main objective.

I slipped it on and glanced in the mirror: long, black dress, extending from the top of my neck down to the very base of my ankles; shiny, bald head; pale, white face; dark black circles surrounding my eyes.

"Who do I look like?" I thought. "Who is it?"

I knew I looked like someone, but I just couldn't place my finger on who it was. A relative? A friend?

Wait ... I know! Sing along with me everyone:

Da, da, da, dum (clap clap)

The house is a museum

Where people come to see 'em

They really are a screa-um

The Addams Family

Of course—Uncle Fester!

I laughed at myself while I took off the dress. Apparently, this wasn't going very well, and I left before I could torment myself anymore.

My sister loaned me one of her dresses. I also wore my wig for the first time at that wedding. I still had a few remaining eyebrow hairs, so I was able to get away with just shading them in a little.

When my eyebrows fell out completely, the only time I drew them on was when I was wearing my wig. When I wore baseball hats, which was most of the time, I never really bothered. I only felt obligated to draw them on when I wore a wig because I thought it looked funny with a full head of hair and no eyebrows.

Then again, I should have thought twice before drawing *anything* on my face. Let me tell you, drawing eyebrows is not as easy as it may seem. You'd be shocked at how much of an impact they have on a person's facial expression. I was never able to get the right arch. My poor attempts at drawing them on always left me looking very "mad" or very "surprised."

I would delicately take the pencil and slowly glide it across my brow bone to achieve just the right arch; however, if my hand swung too high—well, close the lights and duck behind a couch everyone because we're having a surprise party. If my hand swung too low—well, hey jerk, get out of my way. I looked as if I were pissed off at the world!

It was also an adventure when my friend Kate tried to draw my eyebrows for me. I sat on a chair in the middle of her kitchen. She drew and drew, and then drew some more. Pencil, shadow, liner, shadow, pencil ... hell, she might have even thrown some lipstick in there!

After an extremely long time, she had a strange smile on her face as she backed away.

"Okay! I'm done!"

I ran to the bathroom and flipped on the lights. (I should have left the lights off.) I jumped in front of the mirror and saw two slugs sitting above my eyes. I told her what a great job she did and how I loved it, as I scrubbed and scrubbed them away with soap and water.

Margaret also tried to draw my eyebrows.

"What? I think you look so good," she said, as she admired her artwork.

"Sure," I thought. "Maybe for a four-year-old girl, playing dress-up or playing with her mommy's makeup for the first time.

I even tried a makeup artist, which was another disaster. The more everyone tried, the scarier I looked, so most of the time I didn't bother. I was also always too worried that the brows might smudge or run if I started to sweat.

Although I probably should have made more of an effort, any attempt was better than doing nothing. It was something that gave strangers the notion that I was indeed a girl and not a boy wearing a baseball hat.

I began to wear more sporty-looking clothes to go with the baseball hats. My wig was uncomfortable and itchy, and I hated wearing it. It was easier to throw a hat on my head. I went from wearing designer suits, clothes, shoes, and accessories to wearing matching baseball hats and shirts. It became my new trademark. If I was going to be bald and forced to wear a cap, it had to be color coordinated.

One day, when I went to the supermarket, I came across a woman and her three kids. They were standing in the middle of the aisle, and the kids seemed to be giving mommy a hard time. I tried to pass them, but the kids were in my way and I couldn't get through. Realizing this, the woman turned around and yelled at them.

"Will you get out of the way and let the little boy pass!"

I thought, "Huh? Did she just call me a little *boy*?"

Everywhere I turned, I was either "cancer kid," "freak with no hair or brows," or a boy.

A few days before Valentine's Day, my brother Nicholas asked me to go to a senior center with him to help the residents make cards for their families. After we had been cutting, pasting, and coloring paper for some time, an aide wheeled an adorable 102-year-old woman into the room and placed her beside me. (No kidding, she really was 102!)

I was making cards with some of the ladies on my side of the table, and my brother sat directly across from me, helping the others. Not long after the aide wheeled in the 102-year-old woman, I noticed her leaning towards my brother. Lacking discretion, she pointed her finger towards me.

"I don't know what that is," she said with a nearly deaf, 102-year-old effort to whisper.

I politely turned the other way and pretended not to hear her.

"What *what* is?" Nicholas asked.

"What *this* is next to me." Her thumb jerked in my direction. "I don't know if it's a girl or a boy. Whadaya think it is anyway?"

My brother's eyes widened as he realized that she was talking about me!

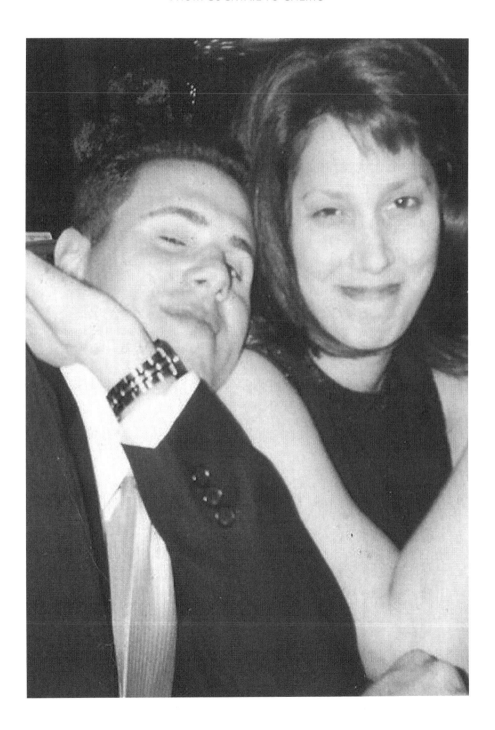

"That's my sister. It's a girl … I mean, *she's* a girl! That's my sister and she's going through chemo right now."

When I was feeling better, I was able to use my baldness to have a little fun. My dad is bald, so I dressed up like him, and then threw a wig on Peter so he could dress up like my mom!

Being bald and wearing just a cap was fun at times, but it also posed problems for obvious reasons that I just mentioned; however, it wasn't all peachy keen wearing my wig either. After a few drinks at my friend's wedding, my wig became the center of attention.

I was dolled up with a dress, makeup, and my wig. The wine I was drinking went right to my head—literally—because I hadn't drunk alcohol in so long, and even a glass or two of wine seemed to get me into a lot of trouble.

It was playtime. I *sneezed* my wig off of my head and into my dinner plate! With every make-believe sneeze I executed, I poked my finger underneath the wig at the crown of my forehead and flipped it off into the chicken. I continued to do this, amusing everyone at my table. Every time my hair would land in my plate, Peter would grab it off the chicken and throw it back onto my head, but it would only stay there long enough until the next sneeze. *Ah-chew!*

There were also times when I had no control over the situation. On one occasion, I went out to dinner with my friends Christine and Billy, wearing my wig. During dinner, I left to go to the bathroom so I could brush it—easier said than done. Apparently, I had put too much gel in it because, with one big swoop, I brushed it right off my head and into the sink.

Naturally, as my luck would have it, the door opened and a lady from the janitorial staff slowly made her way into the bathroom with a cleaning cart. I looked down at my hair in the sink. Without hesitation, I grabbed it and, with both hands, threw it back on top of my head. It may have been messy, crooked, or even lopsided but, most importantly, it was sitting back on my head where it belonged.

The cleaning lady filled the soap dispenser on the other side of the bathroom, and then glanced over at the other dispenser beside me. I gave her an awkward smile from under the untamed animal perched on top of my head. She nodded and managed a phony smile back, but she dared not come close. With her head hanging down and her eyes fastened to the floor, she quickly wheeled her cart across the bathroom and out the door, leaving the animal and me to duke it out.

After taming the angry beast, I went back to the table to tell the tale of "Cleaning Lady Meets Animal."

CHAPTER 14

"Houston, We Have a Problem"

It was time to start the next course of treatment called Taxol, which supposedly wouldn't make me feel as sick; however, I was told that it would most likely give me bone pain, muscle pain, and body aches.

The night before I started this new round of treatment, my cousin, who had another form of cancer and who had previously been on the same type of chemotherapy, called to wish me luck. During our conversation, she warned me to tell my doctor immediately of any problem or difficulty I may encounter when the treatment begins.

The first time the doctor gave her Taxol, *she stopped breathing*.

HOUSTON, WE HAVE A PROBLEM.

Okay. I came this far, and now I was going to die of suffocation.

"Five, four, three, two, one. *Liftoff!*"

I tossed and turned all night, picturing myself being unable to breathe after they gave me Taxol. Naturally, in my world, there wasn't a soul in sight to help me.

I thought, "How long will it take until I *can't* breathe? How long will it take until I *can* breathe? How long will it take until I DIE?"

The next morning, as I sat back in the reclining chair, my mom, my dad, and I waited for my first Taxol treatment. Linda hooked me up to the IV line, and my body was shaking so much that she had to hold down my arm in order to put in the needle.

After the IV line was in place, Linda injected Benadryl into it to prevent any adverse allergic reactions; apparently, Taxol was known to cause allergic reactions. Linda hadn't even pulled the needle out of the IV when the room immediately began spinning around in circles from the Benadryl.

I was terrified *and* dizzy, and now the room spiraled round and round. I felt as if I were on the amusement park ride called the Gravitron, which spins around so fast that you stick to the side of the wall. I clung onto the arms of my chair and squeezed my eyes closed, trying to make it stop. Suddenly, everyone's voice became extremely LOUD and sounded like it was echoing, as if they were projecting their voices through a loudspeaker.

I looked over at Linda, who was preparing the rest of the treatment. She looked blurry, and her entire body was shuddering back and forth as she walked. I took long, deep breaths, just to make sure that I was still breathing.

I looked down at my right arm, positioned straight out onto the armrest. I fixed my eyes on the needle, inserted directly into my arm, and waited anxiously for her to start the Taxol.

Linda shouted, "We're going to begin the Taxol now. Okay, Mary?"

I was disoriented and shaking frantically. I didn't want my mom and dad to see how frightened I was, so I clenched my teeth to try to stop them from chattering. I clutched onto the chair with my other arm to try to stop shaking. I looked down at my legs, which were directly in front of me on the footrest. They, too, were trembling uncontrollably, but I couldn't make them stop.

My mom reached over and held onto my legs. She brushed her hands back and forth, trying to calm me. My entire head and chest were still shaking as I turned to the side and looked the other way. I squeezed my eyes closed just as Linda opened the line. Miraculously, I made it through the first dose without it stopping my breathing, so I continued that treatment once a week for the next three months.

Since I was going to Sloan so often, I made many special friends at the hospital. I knew just about everyone—from the doorman to other patients to volunteers and technicians. Besides my parents and various family members or friends who came with me for my treatments, other patients, technicians, and even cops from Peter's precinct came into the room to sit with me while I was getting my chemo.

Sometimes a group of police cars were scattered outside the Breast Center—all there to keep me company. People passing by the front of the building must have thought there was some big emergency. It looked like an episode of *NYPD Blue*, where all the cops fly up to the front of the building and park in every direction.

I also met Catherine—a 20-year cancer survivor, and one of the very special volunteers. Sue, another patient whom I saw almost every time I went, always kept me laughing. When Sue and I met, she commented on my favorite plaid flannel pants—navy blue, green, and white with yellow stripes. I had bought them in Aruba years ago, and they were the comfiest, craziest-looking pants I had. I loved those pants and often wore them to my treatments. Sue wanted a pair just like mine, and that's how we became friends.

Dr. Andrea, Katherine, and Sandy were so kind and caring. We kept each other laughing, and they continued to pamper me, particularly when new "phantom" cancers—cancers that I had invented or diagnosed all by my smart self—developed constantly.

They'd say, "No, Mary, you don't have cancer in your tooth" or "No, Mary, you don't have cancer in your spleen."

All right. Maybe smart self wasn't so smart after all? Maybe, at the time, all I really needed was a little security and reassurance.

Slowly, as my treatments continued, jokes and magic tricks replaced all of that cancer talk. When I was little, I used to perform magic shows for kids' birthday parties, so I performed magic for the three of them every week. They must have had a lot of patience because they knew exactly how I needed to be treated.

Looking back in retrospect, I realize how, in the middle of their busy day, with a huge room full of people impatiently waiting and complaining, Dr. Andrea, Katherine, and Sandy all stopped what they were doing to watch me perform magic. Not only did they watch, they'd specifically ask for it every time I went to see them.

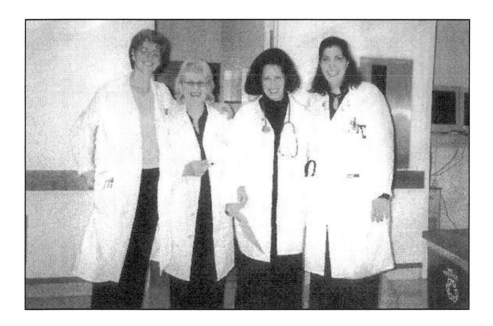

I finally stopped diagnosing myself with different types of cancers, and instead made handkerchiefs float in the middle of the examination room. I thought I was being the "Master of Illusions," but they were getting me to play "magician" instead of "doctor." At one point, I even dressed up like Dr. Andrea and conned my mom into dressing up like Katherine. I was always up to something and kept Dr. Andrea, Katherine, and Sandy on their toes from week to week.

After playtime in the exam room, they would send me back to the waiting room to await my chemo treatment. I remember sitting in the chair and glancing down at my hand. I was being poked and prodded so often that I had bruises on my hand as well as running up and down my arm from the needles.

My skin and nails were turning yellow, and I had terrible muscle and bone pain from the Taxol. It actually hurt to walk. I felt like the Tin Man in need of a good oiling. The pain medication they gave me didn't help very much, and I could barely climb up the stairs. As time went on, I found it difficult to do the simplest things, such as lie in bed and go to sleep.

I would crawl onto my bed, put a pillow under my neck for support, and lie completely still with my arms and legs gently stretched out. I couldn't move any other way. Even the mattress pushing against my bones hurt.

From time to time, I would go for a bone scan, just to make sure there was nothing else going on. I had already convinced myself that the cancer had spread to my bones; when the headaches started, I thought that was cancer, too.

Everything came back normal … no bone cancer! The MRI of my head also came back with nothing on the scan. My family and friends teased me.

"Not even a brain."

The tests and scans continued with my treatments. The more I went, the more tired and sick I became. One day, I sat at the kitchen table while my parents prepared to go out. I felt drained physically and emotionally. As they closed the front door, I leaned onto both of my elbows, wrapped my hands around my bald head, and stared down at the table.

Slowly, my eyes began to well up with tears. They fell one after another, until there was a small puddle resting on the plastic tablecloth in front of me. I didn't move or make a sound as I continued to quietly cry. The only thing I heard throughout the entire house were my teardrops, falling from my face onto the table.

Drip. Drip. Drip.

After a while, I pulled myself out of the chair and stood up. I grabbed onto a few napkins to wipe away the pool of water that had accumulated. Then, I walked up the stairs and crawled into bed.

My blood count deteriorated, and I was in and out of hospitals and emergency rooms throughout the duration of my treatments. By the end, my white blood cell count was so low that I had to give myself injections at home to increase it. To do this, I was supposed to squeeze a little fat together on my leg. (Clearly the easy part—there was plenty of *that* to go around.) The not-so-easy part was actually sticking in the needle.

I could not build up the courage to do it. I looked down at my leg and then looked at the tip of the needle. I swung my hand back and forth, all ready to stick it in, but I just couldn't do it. It's a strange feeling when you have to stab yourself with something.

Mistake #1: I walked into my parents' bedroom and asked my mom to help.

She dashed over to her dresser drawer and pulled out a gigantic magnifying glass.

I gasped.

As she held it in one hand, she grabbed hold of my arm with the other hand and pulled me into their bathroom. I sat down on the toilet seat and glanced up to see my mother leaning over the sink, saying a prayer. Oddly, I didn't run for my life.

I thought, "What was she praying for? That she would be able to do it? That it wouldn't hurt? That she wouldn't jab me in the wrong place?"

Growing up, my mom was never able to see very well, even when I had something as simple as a splinter.

"Oh! I think I *see* it!" she'd say, with the tweezers heading for my finger.

"But Mom, the splinter's in my *foot*!"

Now, she reached over the counter and snatched her eyeglasses. After putting them on and cautiously picking up the syringe, she turned around. She raised the magnifying glass in front of her eyeglasses and held it up to her face. Her eyes were amplified five times the original size through the multitude of glass, and she slowly inched towards me.

"Okay. On the count of three," she said, while swinging her arm into the air and counting aloud. "One. Two. *Three!*" The needle headed directly for my leg. When it was just about to penetrate, she swerved it off to the side. "I can't do it, Mary."

She took a few steps away from me and looked back, and her eyeglasses began to slide down her nose from the perspiration on her face. After another quick prayer, she walked back to me.

"Okay, okay. We can do this."

Mistake #2: I allowed it to happen again.

"Ready. Set. *Go!*"

Her arm jerked back and forth and, after swinging it up and down for some time, she broke down and her eyes filled with tears.

"I just can't do it, honey. I'm sorry. Let's see if your father can."

She opened the bathroom door and called for my dad.

Mistake #3: I allowed my dad to help.

"What do you need?" he shouted while lowering the volume on the TV.

"Ben, we need you to give Mary her injection."

My father got up from the bed and confidently headed into the bathroom. With great certainty, he lifted his pajama pants and rolled up his sleeves, as if he were getting ready for a fight. Then he strolled over to the sink and picked up the needle.

He held it up to the light, and his eyes squinted as he carefully inspected the syringe. It seemed to meet his approval, so he walked over to me, got down on one knee, and leaned in towards my face.

"So you need me to put this in your leg, huh? I'm just supposed to stick it in?"

"Yes, Dad. You can just ... *OW!*"

Without looking away from my face, he stuck the needle into the side of my leg.

"So *that's* how you do it?" he proudly asked, as he handed my mom the needle.

After pinching my cheek and giving me a kiss, he rolled down his sleeves and walked out of the bathroom. Distraction was this wise guy's strategy, and it clearly worked!

The next morning, I woke up with a horrible headache. It was Sunday, so we had to call the emergency room at Sloan. The emergency doctor asked my mother a question.

"So she had breast cancer that spread to her brain?"

"No, no!" my mother shouted, trying to understand his thick accent.

He told her to take my temperature. It was slightly elevated, so he instructed us to come to the hospital immediately. I was devastated.

We arrived in the emergency room where they placed me into a cubicle, sectioned off by curtains, and set up an IV line. A few curtains over, I saw a young man, who was lying in bed and repeating painful noises. After a while, his cries finally ceased.

Not long after that, the ER staff wheeled a woman into the ER on a gurney, wheezing loudly and almost gasping for air. My mom and I looked over at the woman and then back at each other.

I saw my mom's lips move but no words came out, which meant that she was praying. When she lifts her hand up to her chest, makes the sign of the cross over her heart, and then says things under her breath, it always means that she is saying a prayer. She must have been praying for that woman and the many other very sick people who were there that day.

At last, the ER doctor came in and told us that everything was fine. My temperature was down, and the staff didn't believe that I had any bacterial infections. My blood count was a little high, but that was most likely from the injections I was giving myself.

The ER doctor made a gesture with his hands, implying quotations, and said that the "cancer" or the "chemo" can cause different levels in the body to fluctuate.

"Do you think the cancer is back, Doctor?"

He looked down and shook his head.

"No, no. I really don't think so."

That didn't sound very convincing.

Then, the headache was gone for the most part and the fever subsided. The nurses disconnected me from the IV line and I hopped off the bed. I was going home! I said my good-byes to everyone and sprinted out. Peter was outside, talking to my dad, and they both looked over and smiled as I marched through the ER doors.

I finished chemo on November 8th and began the Herceptin infusions directly afterward. Those treatments would continue weekly for the next year—52 treatments in all.

In celebration of finishing the first course, Peter took me out for a special dinner. I got completely dolled up, wig and all, and we headed for Manhattan for a great night out. We were celebrating a tremendous milestone.

I ordered a giant goblet of cabernet, savoring the first sip I took. It had been a very long time since I had wine. As I swallowed, it seemed like the best glass of wine I'd ever had. It was a great dinner, and afterwards we walked along the city streets towards our car.

As we strolled side by side, holding each other's hand, a quiet breeze blew against our faces. I was glowing. I turned to Peter with a great big smile on my face, just about to tell him how happy I was. We both looked at each other and Peter burst out laughing. He was hysterical and barely able to get the words out of his mouth as he pointed at my head.

"Your, your, your, your wi …"

"My *what*?"

"Your wi …, honey!"

"*What?* I can't understand you, Peter."

"YOUR WIG IS COMING OFF!"

My hands quickly flew on top of my head. It was completely bare. As my hands continued backward, I finally met up with my wig, which was hanging off the back of my head.

You would think that, instead of pointing and laughing, Peter would have slid it gracefully back into place, but no. He acted as if it were the funniest thing he had ever seen. Without any help from him, I pushed it back onto the top of my head and held it in place until we reached the car.

When I got home that night, I went straight into my mom and dad's bedroom to tell them about the wonderful time I had. My mom was watching TV when I burst into the room. I immediately began to discuss the fun evening we had. I bragged about the dinner and the magnificent fine wine. It was the first time in months that I was back to my fun, rambunctious old self.

After a lengthy but interesting conversation, I started to walk out the door. My mother quickly sat up in bed and started to get all choked up.

"You're laughing uncontrollably, you're all flushed, and you smell like booze. I am so happy. You're just like yourself again!"

She had never before commended me for coming home drunk. I grunted, gave a baffled look, confused by her praise, and then walked out.

A couple of weeks later, I had surgery to replace the temporary expander in my chest with a permanent implant. They kept me in the hospital one night so they could give me pain medication through my IV. Peter stayed with me and let the Snoring Queen go home.

By morning, I was feeling a little better. Peter and I sat on my bed, waiting for the doctor to come and give the okay to go home. We were discussing the new implant. I pressed it a little and explained what it felt like.

"It still feels like a baseball in my chest."

"It probably just needs time to settle in, Mary."

"You can press on it if you want, Peter. It's not real. Go ahead. It's a little weird though."

Peter's back was towards the door, but he turned around to make sure we had completely closed the curtain around my bed. All embarrassed, he leaned towards me, lifted up his arm, and slowly headed for the mound.

With his hand hovered over my chest, seconds from squeezing it, the curtain flung open. Two doctors stood there, staring back at us in shock. Their clipboards dropped to their sides and they didn't move for an uncomfortable five or 10 seconds.

"Oops, um, sorry. Wrong room," one of them said, and they quickly closed the curtain.

"Wait! No! No! This *is* the right room!" I shouted.

Peter retracted his hand, jumped up, and ran to catch them. I was waiting for a long time that morning to be released, and certainly wasn't about to let them get away on a technicality! After a quick examination, they let me go home, but I still felt the need to explain why my boyfriend's hand was groping my chest.

"No need to explain," they kept saying.

Some things are better left unsaid.

When I got home later that day, I realized that my old, yellow rosary beads were missing. I knew I had brought them to the hospital, as I had every other time, but they weren't in any of my bags and I couldn't find them anywhere.

I had those rosary beads for as long as I could remember—probably since I was four years old. They were big, yellow plastic beads, held together by old string that had begun to turn brown. I had several pins clasped to it: an angel, a dove, and St. Jude.

I always slept with them under my pillow. For many years—prior to my cancer diagnosis—when I was upset or not feeling well, I would fall asleep with the beads clasped tightly in the palm of my hand. I took them with me on every trip. By holding them, I always felt a sense of peace. My sister Margaret borrowed them on her wedding day, and I lent them to friends and family on several occasions, thinking that they would help others to feel the way I did.

Now, my rosary beads came with me through my battle with cancer, so you can imagine how upset I was when I got home from the hospital and saw that they were missing. I called the lost and found, housekeeping, and the nursing station for the floor I was on, with no luck. My rosary beads were gone for good.

My friend Lisa told me that maybe God had planned for someone else to find them, and it was time for them to help that person the same way they helped me. Maybe I didn't need them anymore, and someone out there did.

I was very upset. After I finally settled down, my mom told me that a package had come in the mail for me. I opened it up and found an adorable get-well bear. I tore open the envelope and read the card:

With our deepest sympathy at the time of your loss ...
Love, Kate and Steve

Instead of a get-well card, Kate bought a *sympathy* card for me! There's nothing like accidentally buying your friend with cancer the wrong card. As much pain as I was in, I collapsed off my chair, laughing hysterically with tears running down my face. I immediately called to thank Kate for the gift and the *condolences*.

After we spoke, I went to lie down for a while. Every so often, when I needed to get up from bed, my mom would have to come and lift me. She would put both of her arms underneath my armpits and around to my back to pull me up. When she did this, I would scream out in agony. The pain was like someone stabbing me with a knife into all areas of my chest.

Later that night, I developed a 104-degree fever. I took my temperature in the middle of the night but didn't want to call the hospital to tell them. I knew they'd tell me to come in, and that's the last thing I wanted to do. I didn't tell a soul how high my temperature was and just retreated to my room for the next few days. I continued taking Tylenol to bring the temperature down and bathed in ice-cold water.

The fever subsided and, by Monday, when I called the hospital, they said that my body was most likely adjusting to the implant. As long as the fever was gone, it was okay.

A week and two days after my surgery, my friend Christine was getting married. I was in her bridal party and wouldn't miss the wedding for the world. I proudly walked down the aisle for my friend, despite my pale, clammy body and stitches clinging to my nylon dress. The surgery couldn't have been postponed until after the wedding because I needed time to recuperate before starting radiation treatments.

Before starting radiation, they made a plastic mold of my upper body so that, when I went for treatments every day, all I had to do was lie on the table in that premade body cast. They measured depth, height, and other variations based on my size and the areas they planned to radiate. They needed the precise measurements of my lungs and other organs so the radiation wouldn't come in contact with areas that it shouldn't. The cast put my body in a specific position to guarantee that the radiation would hit the same place every time.

Except for an occasional adjustment here and there, the technicians would place the mold on the table, I would lie in it, and they would flip on the switch. A machine would rotate around the table, directing the beams on the four areas of my body they cited as "at risk" for cancer cells. They did this procedure every day for the next six weeks, with the exception of weekends and holidays.

From the first day, everyone at the hospital made me feel at home ... well, if my home had a radiation machine sitting in the middle of the living room! The technicians who administered the treatments—Jolene, the front desk receptionist, and Dr. Blum—were all very nice. Dr. Blum explained how everything worked and how the staff would take very good care of me.

During my first consultation, I asked her a question.

"If radiation causes cancer, then is it possible for this treatment to actually give me *more* cancer?"

Dr. Blum's frank and straightforward response undoubtedly got the point across to me within seconds.

"Breast cancer is threatening your life, Mary. The chance of this radiation treatment causing more cancer is minimal; however, even if 10 or 15 years down the road it did produce lesions, it will most likely be a less invasive carcinoma. God forbid that ever happened, we would deal with it then. So, for now, this is going to help you, not hurt you."

She also described how the radiation should destroy any remaining cancer cells.

"Hopefully, the Herceptin treatments will take care of anything deeper inside since you do have Level 3 nodes involved."

The Herceptin infusions were the clinical trial for which I would be getting treatments for the next year. She explained how they would direct the radiation near my lung, conceivably debilitating a portion of it.

"However," she continued, "in all likelihood, you won't be able to feel the disparity."

I glanced over at my mom, and saw her twist and turn in her seat. As we drove home that day, I remember looking over at the people who were driving next to us, as I did so often on my trips back and forth to Sloan. I wanted to be like them. I wanted my life back again.

I wanted to be normal.

On December 19th, I walked up to the front desk and checked in with Jolene for my first radiation treatment. Soon after, they called me into the back room. I changed into a gown and they escorted me through the "Hazardous" doors, which had all sorts of warnings written on them.

I lay on the table as Mark, Jackie, Nicole, and some of the other technicians walked in and out of the room. One of them maneuvered a huge machine directly on top of me. They all continued to make small talk, probably to calm me down, but it wasn't working.

"Will it hurt?"

"No, not at all," one responded. "Don't worry. Okay, sweetie?"

When they finally finished setting up, they walked out of the room one by one. Over a loudspeaker, the technicians told me to lie still. I wondered if my quivering body would make a difference—that is technically considered "moving," isn't it?

I looked at the red beam of light aimed directly at me. Suddenly, I heard a very loud buzzing sound, like the kind your clothes dryer makes. Then, all the lights around me flickered and dimmed, as if they were sucking up all the electricity in the hospital just to zap me with radiation. They repeated this procedure four times, as the technicians entered and exited the room to adjust my body and the machine.

We laughed and joked between each session. There was nothing funny about radiation, but we always found something to amuse us. Knowing that they were trying to keep me preoccupied, I'd laugh along with them. Pinned down to the table with a mammoth piece of equipment suspended over me, I figured that, if I can't beat 'em, I might as well join 'em.

After a few weeks, the radiation still didn't hurt, but I had sort of a strange sensation—probably the feeling that food gets after being in the microwave. There's no way to explain it other than it felt as if I were being cooked from the inside out.

One time, when they were setting me up on the table, the measurements didn't seem to make sense. After walking in and out of the room several times, adjusting the machine and me, I heard one of the techs page Dr. Blum. After some discussion, they concluded that the measurement for the depth to my lung had changed.

"Oh, no! I must have *lung* cancer now!" I thought. "The depth changed because there is a tumor in my chest. I just *know* it!"

Contrary to my belief, they told me they thought it was because I was taking deep breaths and hyperventilating.

Hyperventilating? Naturally, I was hyperventilating.

CHAPTER 15

"Goin' to the Chapel and We're Gonna Get Married ..."

W hen I was a little girl, I always dreamed of marrying a tall, dark, and handsome man. I imagined him strong but still caring, sensitive, and fun. Okay, I was like any other little girl ... I dreamed of marrying Mr. Wonderful.

Peter told me some wonderful things early on, when I first got sick.

"Even if you only have six months to live, I will stand by your side and make it the best six months of your life. You're going to outlive *me*, but I still want to cherish our time together."

Christmas Eve was finally here. My mom, my dad, Bernie, and I had plans to go to a restaurant for an early dinner; unfortunately, Peter was working and wouldn't be able to make it. The rest of the family was going to get together the next morning on Christmas Day.

I was still going through radiation treatments and was more tired than usual. I threw on one of my baseball hats and a matching sweater—white was the color of the day. Just as we were walking out the door, my mom turned to me.

"Mary, why don't you wear your wig?"

"I don't really feel like it."

"Dad might want to take some pictures. Why don't you wear it? It'll look nice for the pictures."

I wasn't feeling particularly well and was never comfortable or relaxed wearing my wig anyway. There was always too much drama attached to wearing it. It was extremely uncomfortable, the fibers made my eyes tear, and I always felt as if it were going to fall off.

"What's so important about wearing that stupid wig anyway?" I thought. "She never said anything about wearing my hat before."

I may have been a little touchy at the time since I didn't feel well, so I defended my position.

"Well, if I'm not good enough to be in pictures with my hat on, then maybe I shouldn't be in pictures at *all*?"

"Okay, okay. *Don't* wear the wig, Mary. I just thought it would be nice, that's all."

"Come on, let's go!" my father shouted, as he hurried out the door.

It was an elegant restaurant, beautifully decorated for the holidays. Christmas carolers were strolling amongst the warm fireplaces, singing festive holiday carols. Love and cheer filled each of the many rooms of the restaurant.

My dad was still outside, parking the car, when the maître d' walked over. He escorted us through the first room and into one of the larger rooms in the back. Our table was in the corner, surrounded by a few chairs and a couch, which wrapped around the other side. I sat down on the couch, facing the rest of the room. I looked out at everyone, soaking it all in. Continuing to irritate me, my mother pointed across the table.

"Why don't you sit in *this* chair instead? This chair seems much more comfortable and higher up than that couch you're sitting on now."

I thought, "What is her *problem*?"

"No, I am fine where I am, Mom. I don't feel good, and it really doesn't matter where I sit."

"Okay, okay."

My dad walked into the room and sat down beside my mother. We looked on as one of the carolers strolled over, playing his guitar and singing a Christmas jingle. Everyone watched and smiled. You could smell a mixture of the delicious food, burning wood from the fireplace, and pine from the Christmas trees throughout the restaurant.

We continued to enjoy the evening's festivities but, after the waitress placed our first course down, I casually turned my head and looked across the room towards the door.

I picked up my soda and, as I was taking a sip, I saw a tall gentleman with a headset, wearing a dark black suit, walk through the entry. He was talking into a mouthpiece while weeding his way through the crowd, heading directly towards us. Just as he turned the corner, I spotted Peter behind him.

I thought, "What is going on?"

With an extremely nervous smile, I saw Peter take an enormously deep breath. The clinking glasses and clanking dishes, which were echoing around the room, immediately quieted down. The music stopped, and everyone ended their conversations to turn their head and watch. Peter was accompanied by two gentlemen—one in front of him and one behind him. Confused, I turned to the side and looked at my parents.

"Did he get off of work early to surprise me?" I thought. "What's all the fuss about?"

I glanced back, and the three men were standing face to face with me. Peter shook both of their hands and the other two left.

He was in his full-dress police uniform. Before me stood a gentleman officer, wearing a formal jacket, white dress shirt and tie, hat, white gloves, and shiny black shoes. He extended both arms in front of him, holding a fancy, shiny silver platter. On top of the platter was a small, white box with a red bow, and alongside of it was one red rose.

A beaming grin, reaching from ear to ear, shone across his face. I slowly sunk down into my seat. As I looked up at him with my cap, bald head, and pasty white, sick face, he placed the platter onto the table in front of me. The entire room was watching, anxious to see the ending to this fairy-tale moment.

All of a sudden, I saw Bernie's hand whiz across my face and snatch the box off the platter. She swung it around in the air, like a paper plane.

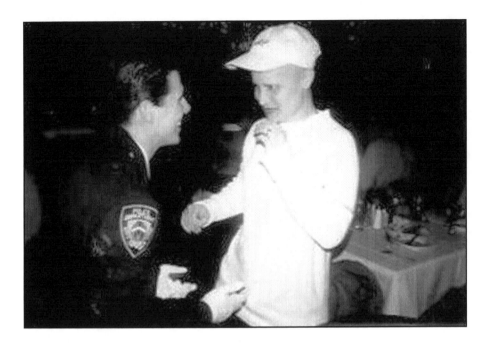

All at once, and all together, my dad, my mom, Peter, and I lunged for her hand.

All at once, and all together, we missed.

Everyone struggled to grab it from her, but she continued dipping, circling it around, and switching hands with it. This amazing romantic moment quickly turned into a struggle as the four of us wrestled with my sister to get the box from her.

"Bernie, give it to me. Give it back, will you? GIVE IT BACK NOW, BERNADETTE!"

She kept giggling and swinging it round and round in the air. Even the waitress dashed for the box. Each time we were just about to snatch it, she'd slyly manipulate it out of reach, leaving our hands grabbing at the air. Finally, Peter was able to get it from her.

After everyone settled down, Peter took me by the hand ever so gently and led me around to the front of the table. He opened up the white box and slowly pulled out a small, black velvet jewelry box. His eyes filled with tears as he took his hat off and placed it under his arm. He carefully opened the box and lowered himself onto one knee.

With tears pouring down his face, he said, "Mary Margaret Stolfa, will you marry me?"

You could hear the entire room collectively inhale and hold its breath. At a time when we were both unsure about the future—even if there were a future at all—we were now courageously taking the very first step towards it.

As I stood there, I thought about the trials and triumphs that brought us to this place—what we lost and what we won. We made it this far and there would be no stopping us now. A serene calmness came over me and I took a deep breath.

My eyes welled up with tears and I said, "Yes. I will marry you, Peter."

The entire room applauded as he slipped the ring onto my finger and I threw myself into his arms.

CHAPTER 16

I Hope You Dance

My hair was slowly growing back and I wore hats on a daily basis as I went for my weekly infusions of Herceptin. As I had been doing all along, I wore a matching hat and shirt. If I wore a red shirt, I'd wear a red hat; if I wore a powder blue shirt, I'd wear a powder blue hat.

At this point, I had a couple of inches of hair sprouting from my head, but I just couldn't give up the hats yet. It almost looked ridiculous to wear one all of the time because I had a full head of hair, but I still couldn't help feeling self-conscious.

One day, my friend Liana, who was my sister Margaret's friend, quickly changed my mind. She had worked with Margaret as a teacher. After hearing about me, and being a breast cancer survivor herself, Liana asked if she could help.

I quickly learned that she was one of the nicest people in the world—so kind, caring, thoughtful, and completely unselfish. I truly believe that people come into our lives for a reason. Whether we get to share one year with them or 50, their time in our lives serves a purpose.

Liana was finishing her chemo treatments the same time I started mine. Throughout that time, she called to see how I was doing. She inspired me with all the love and strength she had.

"Mary, look how well I'm doing. You're going to be just fine, too! You'll make it through just like I did."

They were such encouraging words from such a remarkable person. At times, when I felt as if I wanted to give up, I'd get a call from Liana. Not long after we became friends, she told me that she loved me before hanging up the phone. She had all the love in the world to share and wasn't ashamed to show it. I guess she knew what was truly important in life: to share your feelings with the ones you love because you can never tell someone often enough how much you care.

Unfortunately, by the end of the year and as my treatments continued, Liana learned that her cancer had returned. While on the phone one day, she implied that she had enough and wanted to give up. She said that she didn't think she could take it anymore. That day, we made a pact.

"If I promise you that I won't give up," she said, "will you promise me that you'll stop wearing a hat and show off that hair and face of yours?"

"How could I possibly say no to that?" I thought.

"You have yourself a deal, Liana! Remember, though, you can't give up. Okay?"

I was very upset when I hung up the phone. Even though I knew she had no way of knowing whether I wore my hat, I left the house without it— embarrassed about my hair but proud of my friend. My crooked, lopsided, unshaped hairdo was a huge statement. It didn't mean that I looked ugly; it just meant that my friend wasn't giving up.

Over the next few weeks, Liana became more ill and they admitted her into the hospital. From her hospital bed, she called to tell me how much she loved me and to thank me for everything I had done.

Thank *me*? It shouldn't have been her calling me. It should have been me calling to thank *her* for the 19 months of precious friendship she had so generously given to me. It's amazing how someone can become a part of your life for such a short time and have such a tremendous impact on it. She helped me walk through the roughest time in my life and showed me what it truly means to be courageous.

I kept the promise every day by walking past the pile of hats in my room and leaving them behind. Liana taught me how I now had something much more precious than a pretty haircut: *I had my life.*

She showed me how to be proud and how a person can be her bravest when at her sickest. She never complained about how much pain she was in or how scared she was, even when I visited her in the hospital.

One day, I walked into her room and she patted the bed beside her, gesturing for me to come and sit down. My hair looked horrible, and it was sticking out all over the place but, with a big smile, Liana ever so gently ran her hand through it and told me how proud she was of me. Before I left, I placed a pillow beneath her head and helped tuck her into bed. I gave her a kiss and told her that I loved her.

For some reason, I hesitated before leaving and stopped at the doorway. I turned around and our eyes met and locked, and we gazed at each other for a minute. I lifted my hand up and waved good-bye.

That was the last time I saw Liana alive.

I found out the following week that she lost her battle with cancer. I knew how she bravely fought to keep her promise and not give up, and I could not have been prouder of her.

She gave me a tremendous amount of strength during our short-lived friendship. From then on, as my crooked haircut continued to shape and grow long again, I would walk outside, look up at the sky, and brush my hand through my hair.

"See, Liana? I kept my promise. I'm not giving up either."

A year and a half after I had walked in for my first chemo treatment with my body shaking, I marched through those very same doors with unfathomable emotion.

This would be my last treatment.

For the past couple of years, I had endured numerous surgeries, six months of chemotherapy, 28 days of radiation, and a full year of weekly Herceptin infusions. Today, I soared with my wings stretched out wide, like a flying eagle. It was one of the most monumental, invigorating, and proud moments of my life.

I was emotionally empowered but physically weak. The treatments had become somewhat toxic and made my body ache all over. My head, neck, chest, ribs, arms, and legs were sore with each step I took, but this would be a triumphant victory.

I paced myself as I put one foot in front of the other. I may have been hurting but, most importantly, I was still here—standing on my own two feet. My parents and I greeted the doorman and the front desk clerk, our eyes sparkling and our smiles gleaming.

"Hi, J.R. Hi, Jake!"

We exited the elevator onto the lower concourse floor, which was the Breast Center.

"Hi, Asia," I said to the receptionist.

After I met and greeted the staff and patients, as I did every week, Sandy opened up the back door to where the examining rooms were and called my name. She had a huge smile on her face and looked at me with such pride and gratification. With a beaming smile, I walked through the door and into an examination room for the last checkup before my final treatment.

After waiting in the room for a while, Dr. Andrea, Katherine, and Sandy walked in together. They closed the door behind them and stared at me for a good 10 seconds.

"Is something wrong?" I thought.

I may have been cancer free, but I was still suffering from paranoia. Throughout my treatments, I always thought that something was wrong. If they said I was doing okay, I wondered why they didn't say I was doing great. I would always smile and laugh along with them but, even when they smiled and laughed, I thought that they weren't doing it enough. I was always an analytical person, but I gave "analyze" an entirely new meaning when I became sick.

After a brief pause, Katherine swung her hands around from behind her back. As I sat on the examining table, the three of them walked up to me and and pulled out two big bushels of yellow roses and a card.

"Congratulations!" they all cried out.

We kissed and hugged in an emotional celebration. It was extremely moving for me to thank the people who helped save my life. We reminisced and talked about the past, as if we were old friends. Then, the three of them said how it will be sad that we weren't going to be together anymore.

"I know. It's sad, isn't it?" I agreed.

"What are we going to do now?"

I rolled my eyes.

"Come on, guys! It's not like I'm *never* going to see you again. I'll be here in three months for my follow-up exam, and then every three months for a long time after that!"

They glanced at one another with a bewildered look on their faces as they listened to my explanation.

"Wait a minute. Yeah, I guess you're right. Of course we'll see each other!"

Then we all burst out laughing again.

After receiving my last treatment, I said my good-byes to all the people who were so good to me every time I was there. The automatic doors opened, and I left the building that day a completely different person than I had been a year and a half before.

For weeks after, I celebrated with cakes, dinners, cocktails, and several parties with family and friends. My friend Maureen had a party for me at her house. We all gathered around in a circle, as Peter and I stood next to each other, ready to give a toast.

I lifted my glass high and thought about what I had gone through: being sick, having chemo, and enduring many surgeries and heartache. I knew that, no matter how hard I would want to try, I would always remember and never forget what happened. Perhaps there was a reason that I was *supposed* to always remember and never forget.

Even with the cancer spreading to so many lymph nodes, I reminded myself of how I couldn't predict my life based on textbook statistics. None of my doctors ever told me my prognosis and, quite honestly, I really didn't want to know. I refuse to look back and have to say "I should have" or "I could have."

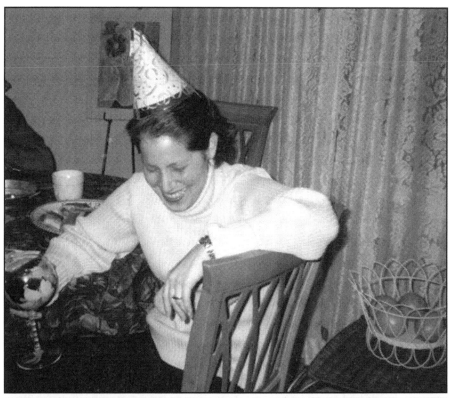

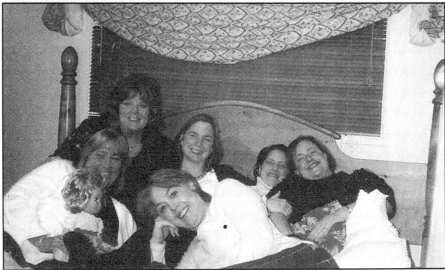

Whether I succeed or fail, I want to be able to say that I tried. Whether I live one more year or 50 more years, I now live to make the best of each day. Fifty years of life doesn't necessarily mean 50 years of living.

I truly believe now that it is the *quality* of life, not the *quantity*. I'm going to take each day as it comes and not sweat the small stuff. Life's too short for that. If I knew in advance about the phone call that I would be receiving on the evening of March 1st, I would have spent all of my time waiting to get cancer.

I never would have had all the vacations, dinners, parties, laughs, and fun. I never would have gone parasailing, jet-skiing, snowboarding, and horseback riding. I never would have *lived*. Cancer may not have taken my life away physically, but it would have taken it from me in so many other ways. I decided not to live my life waiting for another horrible phone call because that call may never come.

How can you focus on living if you're too busy focusing on dying?

When I first got cancer, my sister Margaret gave me a Lee Ann Womack CD. She wanted me to concentrate on the lyrics to the song entitled "I Hope You Dance." I played that song over and over all the time I was sick. I paid close attention to the words, as if it were my sister saying them to me—particularly during times when I wanted to give up (and there were many of those).

I came home from Maureen's party and walked up the stairs to my bedroom. After getting cleaned up for bed, I turned on my stereo, pressed the CD button, hit "Play," sat down on my bed, and listened:

I hope you still feel small when you stand beside the ocean

Whenever one door closes I hope one more opens

Promise me that you'll give faith a fighting chance

And when you get the choice to sit it out or dance

I hope you dance

I hope you never fear those mountains in the distance

Never settle for the path of least resistance

154

Give the heavens above more than just a passing glance

And when you get the choice to sit it out or dance

I hope you dance

I smiled and thought of the many times I wanted to give up. I wanted to take the path of least resistance and sit it out, but I didn't.

I stood up and danced. I had to for many reasons. One of the most important ones would come to surface years later. Exactly 10 years after my diagnosis, Margaret was diagnosed with breast cancer. I was going to have to be here to show her how to dance.

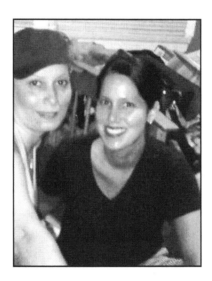

CHAPTER 17

The Mary Stolfa Cancer Foundation

Jesse believed in the concept of "pay it forward." I became friends with Jesse after Dr. Derini asked her to call me when I received my diagnosis. She was a member of a support group and was closest to my age. She "paid it forward" and helped others as they had helped her.

Paying it forward can move mountains, but how could I help and pay it forward? What could I do? How could I give back even a small portion of what others gave me? Could I help others going through the same thing? Can I, somehow, help in some way to find a cure for this dreadful disease?

As a little girl, over a decade and a half earlier, I had begun my crusade, but it hadn't gotten very far. I was all grown up now, but I was still living in a world with cancer. As an adult, I was truly able to comprehend the magnitude of it all.

A man in a white lab coat was not going to find a cure. The encyclopedia at my library would not give me all the answers. The two fundraisers I had as a child (which, at the time, I didn't even know were called "fundraisers") raised only spare change for "research" and wasn't quite enough to find a cure.

Today, we are able to transplant organs and travel from the deep seas into the great outer space, but we still can't stop one damn cell from growing. So how can one person help? How can one person do something to stop this disease from taking so many lives? How can one person help to really, truly, and undeniably make a difference?

In May 2002, the Mary Stolfa Cancer Foundation was born. On my computer, I listed types of cancers from A to Z with informational charts. I also collected "Stories of Hope" for inspiration and a "Wall of Honor" for the ones who lost their battle.

I launched the Mary Stolfa Cancer Foundation website a few months later, giving thousands of people access to information. I introduced several programs, such as the "Hope Program" to assist cancer patients financially, send them on trips, and grant wishes for them during rigorous treatments.

I initiated a "Medication Assistance Program" to pay for chemotherapy when patients could not. I also instituted a "Wig Program" to supply wigs to those unable to afford them, and a "Face-It, You're Beautiful Program" to give a day of beauty to patients undergoing treatments.

I mailed out newsletters, offered support and encouragement to patients, and spoke to audiences about cancer-related issues.

Months later, as I was cleaning out some things from my parents' attic, I came across a box filled with books and papers. I placed the box on the floor and opened it.

I stopped when I spotted an old folder, which had a portion of the top bent backwards. I pushed away the pile of papers scattered on top, picked up the folder, and then placed it down on my lap.

Glued-on letters out of white construction paper reading C-A-N-C-E-R were diagonally across the front of the folder, and I stared at it for a minute. Finally, I opened the folder. The index was scribbled with a marker on the old, yellowing first page—"Cancers from A to Z"—and a list of cancers followed: "Bladder Cancer, Brain Cancer, Breast Cancer ..."

It was the report that I made back in elementary school. Looking at it now, I realized how it was actually the blueprint to my foundation and website.

My battle began back then and now, over a decade and a half later, it had turned into a full-blown war. Once again, I gathered my friends to raise money. Everyone came together for the very first Mary Stolfa Cancer Foundation fundraiser.

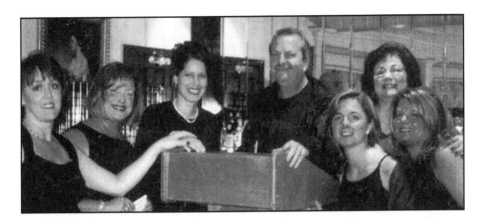

At my elementary school, we had sold greeting cards outside the gym on the day of the show to raise funds for cancer. Now, just before this first fundraiser for the foundation, someone introduced me to a very special woman named Debra. After losing her friend of 25 years to breast cancer, Debra had created her own line of beautiful greeting cards for people going through cancer and set up her display of cards.

We sold tickets for weeks leading up to the fundraiser, and history seemed to be repeating itself. The hall was jam packed, and I stood off to the side of the stage and waited for my call to the podium.

In that moment, I felt like a child again, wearing a costume from one of those shows back in elementary and junior high schools: oversized dress-up pants, with the legs dragging down past my feet and onto the floor; my dad's big shirt, hanging off my shoulders, with the tips of my fingers barely peeking out from the extra-long sleeves, and scuffed up sneakers. As I looked at the audience from the side of the stage, it was as if I were looking through the eyes of that determined little girl.

I heard my friend Randy call my name, so I slowly began to walk towards him. With each step I made towards center stage, I "shed" one piece of that child's costume at a time and grew into the woman I had become. My first step left the dress-up pants behind; the second step dropped the giant shirt; with the last step, I lost the sneakers.

Now, wearing a beautiful, long black dress and high heels, I stood before the audience. My hair was done up and I wore makeup and jewelry. My dress had

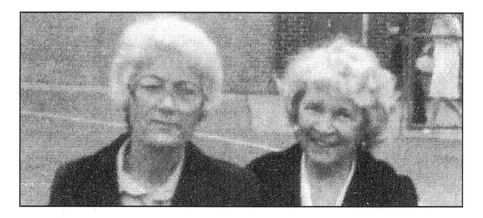

straps around my shoulders and dipped down in the front; beneath it, cancer scars ran across my chest. I looked out into an audience filled with hundreds of people.

This time, little faces from elementary and junior high school were not looking back at me nor were the faces of Mrs. Sheery, Mr. Hildebrandt, or any of my other teachers. This time, family, friends, and strangers had all come together for the same reason.

As I stood there and looked at them, I explained how each of us should always remember that there is "hope for the future." In spite of what happened to me, my friends, and my family because of cancer, I knew that both of my grandmothers would have agreed. I also knew that, in some way, both were out there in that sea of faces: one wearing her "crooked cookie glasses"; the other holding onto that dressy white communion sock—both smiling back at me.

As I continued to speak, I explained how money raised for the foundation would go towards ... *cancer research.*

CHAPTER 18

"My Boobies Went to Heaven"

After having cancer, I found myself spending a lot of time thinking about why things happen and how they must happen for a reason. Over the years, friends and family were diagnosed with cancer. Some lost. Some won. Some are still fighting.

Perhaps one of the reasons I got sick was to help those loved ones who were diagnosed.

Perhaps it was to institute my foundation and continue the mission I started so many years ago.

Perhaps it was to protect my sister Bernadette from cancer. Because of one of my tests, we later found out that Bernie also carries the same breast/ovarian cancer gene as Margaret and I. The doctors recommended to electively have her breasts and ovaries removed to prevent her from getting either cancers. I wish all of us could have been as brave as Bernie. After her surgery, she told everyone, "My boobies went to heaven."

Maybe everything in life *does* happen for a reason.

Over time, my sickness continued to teach me many lessons, and one was extremely significant and valuable. From the time of my diagnosis, I started to look at the world in a completely different way.

I learned to reevaluate my priorities and gain a better understanding of what "really" matters. Before I got sick, I had taken each day and each person who was part of my life for granted. I didn't share my feelings with loved ones as often as I should have. I always thought that I had "tomorrow" to say, "I love you."

160

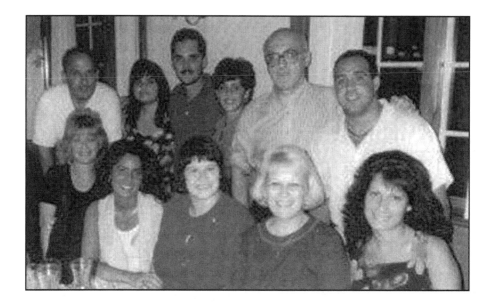

I learned that we should tell each other how we feel *before* we get sick or *before* we die. In this way, we live knowing how much we're loved, and not die eventually finding it out.

Before I had reached age 30, it took something like cancer to show me what I should have known all these years. Cancer taught me my answer to the age-old question, "What is the meaning of life?" It's ironic how something can rob us of life and teach us a significant and poignant lesson about it at the same time.

Love.

There is nothing greater in this world than that amazing, warm feeling you get inside when you love someone or know that someone loves you. Regardless of how rich or poor—and sick or healthy—you are, no one and nothing can take that away from you … not even cancer.

I realized that life wasn't about being rich with expensive cars, clothes, or homes. It was about being rich with family and friends, cherishing and appreciating the time I have with each of them instead of letting each day pass me by. The family has grown a lot since the time when this photo was taken and I was sick.

I don't know what happens when we die—although I do have my thoughts about it—but I'm almost positive that we don't take our "things" with us. I'll bet everything I own that the one thing we *do* take with us is the love we have and share. You can never tell someone often enough how much you care. I know that now because not everyone gets a second chance.

Life is a wonderful gift, and it truly is a *gift*, not a free give-away. Every laugh, every tear, every smile, every breath, and every day I can share with the people whom I love is a precious gift from God. I thank Him for it every chance I get.

In a world filled with many doubts, uncertainties, and fears, where people can step out of your life just as easily and quickly as they step in, there is so much good that life has to offer—excitement and dreams of what today has in store for us, and what tomorrow may bring. Love, hope, and faith will always help us find our way.

A good friend of mine once said to me, "This too shall pass." If we can remember that, particularly when everything else in the world seems to be going wrong and we think we can't do it, we'll come to realize that we will get past it all ... even if, at the moment, it seems like there is no end in sight.

Although I'll never be the same person I was before I had cancer, when I turn my head to look back on what happened to me, I realize how much I have learned and how strong it has made me.

No matter what crosses our path, there is always a wish fulfilled, a prayer answered, and a cocktail at the end of the tunnel.